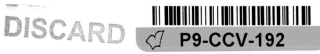

4/14

CAFFEINATED

CAFFEINATED

How
OUR DAILY HABIT
HELPS, HURTS, *and*
HOOKS US

MURRAY CARPENTER

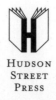

HUDSON
STREET
PRESS

HUDSON STREET PRESS
Published by the Penguin Group
Penguin Group (USA) LLC
375 Hudson Street
New York, New York 10014

USA | Canada | UK | Ireland | Australia | New Zealand | India | South Africa | China
penguin.com
A Penguin Random House Company

First published by Hudson Street Press, a member of Penguin Group (USA) LLC, 2014

REGISTERED TRADEMARK—MARCA REGISTRADA
HUDSON
STREET
PRESS

ISBN 978-1-59463-138-2

Printed in the United States of America
10   9   8   7   6   5   4   3   2   1

Set in Bell Regular
Designed by Eve L. Kirch

To my parents, Chuck and Sally Carpenter

Contents

PART III. CAFFEINATED BODY, CAFFEINATED BRAIN

PART IV. CORRALLING CAFFEINE

Introduction:
A Bitter White Powder

Propped up on my desk before me, there is a vacuum-sealed Ziploc bag of white powder. About the size of a compact disc, the package weighs one hundred grams. The powder is an alkaloid, extracted from the leaves and seeds of plants that grow at mid-elevations in low latitudes.

Chemists would recognize this substance as a methylated xanthine, composed of tiny crystalline structures. Biologically, the molecule is so useful that it emerged independently on four continents as an insecticide, keeping pests from nibbling on its host plants.

Let's get personal—this substance courses through my veins as I write these words. It is a drug, and I have been under its influence nearly every day for the past twenty-five years. And I am in good company. Most Americans take this drug daily. It is so effective, yet so simple, that if it did not grow on trees a neurochemist would have invented it.

This is, of course, caffeine, a bitter white powder. It is the essence of coffee or tea and the key ingredient in soft drinks, energy drinks, and energy shots. In moderation, caffeine is best known for something it does simply and effectively: It makes us feel good. But it is a drug whose strength is consistently underestimated. A sixty-fourth of a teaspoon, the amount in many soft drinks, will give you a subtle boost.

A sixteenth of a teaspoon, about the amount in twelve ounces of coffee, is a good solid dose for a habituated user. A quarter teaspoon will lead to bodily unpleasantness—racing heart, sweating, and acute anxiety. A tablespoon will kill you.

Three years ago, when I decided to follow caffeine where it led me, I thought the drug was fantastic. Not only was it the easiest, cheapest way to rev up my day, increase my concentration, and boost my productivity; I felt sure that it must not be really bad for you (if it were, science would have revealed it by now) and that the industry must be pretty big. But as the story took me to the coffee farms of central Guatemala, the world's largest synthetic caffeine factory in China, an energy shot bottler in New Jersey, and beyond, I learned that I had underestimated caffeine on all accounts.

I had underestimated the drug's effects on our bodies and brains. I had underestimated the scope and scale of the caffeine industry. And I had underestimated the challenges regulators face in trying to rein in an industry running wild.

⚡

Caffeine sharpens the mind, especially for people who are stressed, tired, or sick, whether they use it regularly or not. It was a neuroenhancer long before the term came into vogue. It does not just increase acuity; it can also improve mood. A review of the psychological effects of caffeine puts it this way: "There is ample evidence that lower doses of caffeine are reliably associated with 'positive' subjective effects. . . . The subjects report that they feel energetic, imaginative, efficient, self-confident, and alert; they feel able to concentrate, and are able to work but also have the desire to socialize."

Athletes using caffeine are stronger and faster than their drug-free peers. It has even helped Navy SEAL recruits perform better during the tryouts known as Hell Week, perhaps the most diabolical, arduous test of mental and physical fortitude ever devised. And it's an effective treatment for hangovers.

Caffeine can make you stronger, faster, smarter, and more alert, but it is not quite the perfect drug. In some people, it can trigger severe and unpleasant psychological effects, such as acute anxiety and even panic attacks. These are most pronounced in people with genetic variants that make them more susceptible to caffeine. Any caffeine user who believes it's totally benign should try going without it for a few days. Caffeine withdrawal is real and unpleasant, often including headaches, muscle pain, weariness, apathy, and depression. On a subtler level, many Americans fall into a routine of diminished sleep followed by large doses of caffeine—a vicious circle.

Caffeine is not as powerful as cocaine, which can be deadly at just over a gram in inexperienced users. You'd need to slam about fifty cups of coffee at once, or two hundred cups of tea, to approach a lethal level of caffeination. But if you go straight for the powder, you can get a lot in a hurry. On April 9, 2010, Michael Bedford was at a party near his home in England. He ate two spoonfuls of caffeine powder he'd bought online, washing them down with an energy drink. He soon began slurring his words, then vomited, collapsed, and died. Bedford likely ingested more than five grams of caffeine. The coroner cited caffeine's "cardiotoxic effects" as the cause of death.

The caffeine conundrum is this: It can be a fantastic drug—one of the very best—but, like any powerful drug, it can cause problems with real consequences.

So, it's safe to say that I had definitely underestimated the drug's psychomotor effects. But to a greater degree, I had underestimated the scope and scale of the caffeine industry. I learned that the addictive, largely unregulated drug is everywhere—in places you'd expect it (like coffee, energy drinks, teas, colas, and chocolate) and in places you wouldn't (like orange sodas, vitamin tablets, and pain relievers).

I learned that brands such as Coca-Cola have ducked regulatory efforts for decades, even as they quietly use the drug to reinforce our

buying patterns. I learned that consumers are uninformed about caffeine because Coca-Cola, Monster, 5-hour Energy, and even Starbucks
persistently and systematically downplay the drug's importance.

We need to look no further than the items on my shelf to get a
sense of the breadth of the industry: Amp energy gum, 6 Hour
Power energy shots, and Jitterbeans "highly caffeinated" candy. Cans
of Red Bull, Rockstar 2X Energy, and Mega Monster energy drinks.
There are bottles of Mountain Dew and Coke, and the cans of Diet
Coke and Diet Pepsi that I used to methodically wean myself from
caffeine for the first time in decades. There is a small package of
roasted and ground cacao, which I purchased in Chiapas, where it is
grown. I've got a bottle of Lipton iced tea and a couple of bags of
Morning Thunder, a combination of black tea and yerba maté (an
evergreen South American plant with caffeinated leaves). I've got a
box of black tea packaged by a one-man gourmet tea shop in the
Green Mountains of Vermont and a single-serving K-Cup full of
coffee that was processed in the massive factory a half mile away.
There's a canned coffee drink of the sort that is wildly popular in
Japan and several packs of military-strength chewing gum that I
picked up at an army research lab. There is a package of Starbucks
instant coffee labeled in Mandarin and several ounces of Iron Buddha loose-leaf tea I bought at the world's largest tea market in Beijing. In Ziploc bags, I've got raw kola nuts—the sort that African
men chew for a caffeine boost—and guarana berries, from the South
American vine that packs more caffeine per ounce than any other
plant. There are caffeinated energy gels, too, made for athletes: Clif
Shot Bloks and a foil package of Gu that I picked up at the Ironman
World Championship in Hawaii.

It's worth noting that most of the packages are empty. The energy
shot fresh off the bottling line in New Jersey, the boxes of caffeinated
gel strips and chewing gum, the Java Monster and Rockstar Roasted
coffee-flavored energy drinks, and so on. As it happens, I am an omnivorous and enthusiastic caffeine user.

There have been a few red flags along the road. When I found my-self ordering a batch of cold-pressed, vacuum-extracted coffee con-centrate known as Black Blood of the Earth, I should have known my investigation was veering toward the ridiculous. And when the stuff arrived in test tubes, with its promise of forty times the caffeine of straight coffee, my only thought was, "Hey, this might be really good." You'll also find the empty test tubes there on my shelf (it tasted just fine, when diluted as suggested and consumed in tiny doses).

Then, too, there is the coffee I am drinking now, with milk, from a jelly jar. I brewed it from Colombian beans roasted here in Waldo County just last week. I ground them in a hand-cranked grain mill at five this morning, dumped the grounds into a cone filter, drenched them in hot water, and swilled my first cup with the expectant delight so many of us know so well.

Like most caffeine addicts, I am inclined to believe my primary in-terest is the caffeine delivery mechanism I favor—coffee, in my case. Others have their own favorites. "I love Diet Pepsi," one might say, or, "I am addicted to Starbucks cappuccinos." What few of us are willing to admit is that the essence of our longing is this bitter white powder. But this is natural. Who wants to admit to being addicted to any drug, or even just passionately enthusiastic about it? And make no mistake, despite its ubiquity and apparently benign nature, caffeine is a drug. And it is more powerful and more effective than most of us realize.

Caffeine is not a quirky component of coffee, tea, colas, and energy drinks, but the sine qua non. Scientists have understood for decades that as little as thirty-two milligrams of caffeine, less than the amount in twelve ounces of Coke or Pepsi, significantly improves vigilance and reaction time; many people can detect doses half that size.

If a product delivers a psychoactive dose of a drug that reliably improves mood, alertness, and energy levels, it is reasonable to as-sume that this drug effect is the key attraction. (It would be far more challenging to argue the opposite: that a drug that makes you feel good and is present in psychoactive doses is somehow not a part of the product's allure.)

If we distill all of these products—the coffee, the colas, the energy shots—to their essences, we can see them for what they are: convenient, stigma-free vessels for funneling caffeine into the human body. At the end of the day, they are Caffeine Delivery Mechanisms, or CDMs.

Let's consider that stigma bit, just briefly. As an indication of our conflicted feelings about the drug that is caffeine, consider these scenarios. If a coworker said, "Wow, I am beat. I am going to grab a cup of coffee," it would seem well within societal norms. You might ask her to grab one for you, too. But if the same friend said she was fried, then drew from her pocket a cellophane pouch of white powder, measured off a sixteenth of a tablespoon, and lapped it up or stirred it into a glass of water, it would seem a bit creepy—the sort of thing you might have expected of William Burroughs.

It is fortunate for Coca-Cola, Starbucks, and 5-hour Energy that we consider the latter to be strange behavior, because that is how they have made their millions: by normalizing and adding value to caffeine.

⚡

Talking about caffeine is challenging, partly because we typically speak imprecisely; we don't have a good vocabulary for it. When someone inquires about our caffeine habits, we tend to reply in terms of how many cups of coffee we drink daily. But this a wildly inadequate measure. One five-ounce cup of coffee—the size that has been often used in studies of caffeine consumption—could have less than sixty milligrams of caffeine, while one sixteen-ounce cup could have nearly ten times as much, but both could legitimately be considered one cup of coffee. Catherine the Great used a pound of coffee for her daily five cups, which is clearly on the extreme end of really strong coffee. So if you say you drink three cups of coffee daily, it does not go a long way toward quantifying your caffeine intake.

In an effort to make this easier, I came up with a measure called a Standard Caffeine Dose, or a SCAD. A SCAD is seventy-five milligrams. This is a handy standard, roughly equal to a shot of espresso, five ounces of coffee, one 8.4-ounce Red Bull, two cans of Coke or Pepsi, a sixteen-ounce Mountain Dew, or a twenty-ounce Diet Coke (which has higher caffeine concentrations than Coke).

Normalizing quantities makes it easier for us to understand caffeine doses and learn to use the drug most effectively. For example, I take about four or five SCADs daily. On a two-SCAD day, I will feel slow; on a seven-SCAD day, jittery. So throughout the book, when I reference caffeine content in milligrams, I will also include the content in SCADs, which I hope you will find useful.

Another note on nomenclature: Depending on whom you ask, the consistent daily use of caffeine is a dedicated habit, a physical dependence, or an addiction. I have chosen to use the words *addictive* and *addiction* to describe caffeine's effects and our habits. Obviously, these words are emotionally charged, so I want to be clear that I mean "addictive" in the layperson's sense: People who are habitual caffeine users feel compelled to continue taking the drug and feel lousy when they skip it. What I don't mean to imply is any of the antisocial characteristics often associated with drug addictions—missing work due to a hangover, knocking over a Rite Aid in search of pills, or haunting the seedy parts of town seeking an illicit fix.

⚡

Focus long enough on caffeine, as I have, and you might start to see the world through a caffeine-centric lens. It can be unsettling. On a trip to Houston to learn about powdered caffeine, I picked up a small bag of crude caffeine extracted from coffee. And I started to see products made with powdered caffeine everywhere. I wandered past a tall mural of Big Red and Sun Drop—regional caffeinated soft drinks—in the shadow of the Astros' stadium, Minute Maid Park. At the time, Minute Maid (which is a Coca-Cola company) was producing a caffeinated juice drink. When I stopped for a cup of coffee at a natural foods store in the area, the man sitting at a nearby table was swilling a twenty-ounce Diet Coke. And as I strolled down Walker Street, a pair of attractive brunettes in a Nissan Cube emblazoned with the 5-hour Energy logo came cruising slowly along in the right lane, handing out free samples like inner-city crack dealers trying to get people hooked. You'll find the vial they gave me on my shelf with all the other empty containers.

On my way downtown, I witnessed a strange vignette. A Coca-Cola truck was unloading at the curb. I stopped to take a picture, thinking of the juxtaposition of the crude caffeine in my hand and the finished product. As the truck left the curb, it pulled out sharply into traffic just ahead of a much smaller, older truck that had to brake suddenly, prompting the driver to lean on his horn. It turned out to be a coffee distributor's truck. This scene seemed like the perfect metaphor for the past seventy years of caffeine in America.

The two biggest American caffeine stories of the past seventy years are these: Coffee consumption plummeted, and soft drink consumption soared. In 1975, soft drinks passed coffee as America's favorite beverage and never looked back. Eight of the nation's top ten soft drinks are caffeinated. Soft drink sales have been led by Coca-Cola, the Atlanta company that grew into the world's best known brand. If you put all the Coke ever produced into eight-ounce bottles and stacked them up lengthwise, they would reach to the moon and back more than two thousand times. Worldwide, people consume nearly twenty thousand Coca-Cola beverages per second; that's 1.7 billion daily.

Coca-Cola owes its success to caffeine. Its early formulation had eighty milligrams of caffeine per eight-ounce serving—exactly the same amount as an 8.4-ounce can of Red Bull—and it was marketed as a pick-me-up. That was in 1909, when the federal government first tried and failed to corral the emerging caffeine economy, leaving an astonishing regulatory vacuum that persists to this day.

This brings us to other aspects of caffeine that I'd underestimated:

the regulatory confusion surrounding the substance in America and the dissonance that exists as the FDA tries to figure out when to treat it as a drug and when to treat it as a food. The FDA has long practiced a dual regulatory role for caffeine—regulating it when it's packaged as an over-the-counter medication and mostly ignoring it when it's blended into drinks or labeled as a dietary supplement.

Consider the one-hundred-gram packet of pure caffeine on my desk—ten lethal doses that fit easily in the palm of my hand. I bought it online, with no inquiry about my age or how I intended to use it. It does carry warning labels ("WARNING: Caffeine is HIGHLY TOXIC in large quantities. Improper use may result in death."), but they are not required by law. That is because it is clearly labeled as a dietary supplement, not a drug.

There's yet another CDM here on the shelf in my office—a pill bottle with ninety 200-milligram Jet-Alert caffeine caplets. Like No-Doz or Vivarin, these tablets are regulated by the FDA as over-the-counter drugs and carry this warning on the label: "Limit the use of caffeine-containing medications, foods, or beverages while taking this product because too much caffeine may cause nervousness, irritability, sleeplessness, and occasionally, rapid heartbeat."

But the new generation of energy products that are sort of like energy drinks without the water—gums and gel strips and even handy, Tic Tac–size containers of caffeine powder—seem finally to have caught the agency's attention. As I was completing the writing of this book in May 2013, the FDA announced its investigation of the use of caffeine in this new generation of caffeinated products.

The regulators should definitely pack a lunch and make a day of it. It is always easier to prevent a product from going to market than it is to yank one that's well established, so the FDA is playing catch-up. Corralling caffeine at this point won't be easy. It is the most popular, least regulated drug in the United States and simultaneously the food additive that allowed a product made by a small Georgia company to become the world's best known brand. Caffeine deserves more respect—both for its psychoactive power and for its primary role in American culture—and consumers deserve better regulation and more information.

My quest to understand caffeine has led me to some unlikely places. One of them was a sultry corner of coastal Mexico, where caffeine culture took root thousands of years ago. And that is where this story begins.

PART I

TRADITIONAL CAFFEINE

CHAPTER 1

The Cradle of Caffeine Culture

The pyramids at Izapa were not as spectacular as I had expected. They are low, stone-sided mounds of earth rising beside the main highway to Mexico City, a dozen miles outside of Tapachula, Chiapas. Diesel-spewing buses passed, stirring the plastic detritus at the roadside. A few sad roadhouses tried to capitalize on the location, but business was slow. A local family served as caretakers, selling Cokes and postcards from their porch and charging a small fee to wander the ruins. Roosters crowed from the nearby houses, pigs ambled down a dirt road, and as evening fell, the surrounding woods were full of birdsong.

Called the Soconusco region, this low, flat coastal plain along the Pacific Ocean is torrid—sweltering and rainy. The Soconusco is the birthplace of chocolate culture. The shaded lower tier of the woods that envelop the clearing, which is no more than five acres, is full of cacao trees, just as it has been for much of the past three thousand years.

The people who built these pyramids came after the Olmec and before the Maya. They were so unique that their culture is called Izapan, after this, the best known of their sites. In addition to ancient ball courts and public plazas—like the one at the center of this site—they left behind this tradition of cacao (pronounced kuh-cow). Farmers have been planting and nurturing cacao trees here ever since. This is the tree that grows the bean that gives us chocolate.

An archaeological dig at the nearby Paso de la Amada turned up traces of chocolate more than thirty-five hundred years old. This is the earliest evidence of the human use of chocolate, which in itself is kind of cool, but it's more than that. It is also the earliest documented human use of caffeine. So far, no place on the planet can claim longer continuous caffeine use.

It is tempting to think of chocolate as a modern luxury, an indulgence of self-proclaimed chocoholics. But even the most devoted of today's chocolate lovers have nothing on the Izapans, Mayans, and Aztecs. They really loved their chocolate. They used it ceremonially, in rituals that sometimes included human sacrifice. They drank it spiked with chili and used special pitchers decorated with fierce faces to pour it from high above the cup, giving the chocolate a frothy head. They even used the little cacao beans as currency. The Aztecs rationed it to their soldiers.

During colonization, when chocolate became popular among the courts of Europe, Soconusco chocolate was a favorite among royal chocolate freaks like Cosimo III, the Grand Duke of Tuscany. In 1590, not long after chocolate made its way to Spain and Italy, a Jesuit author noted that the Spanish, and especially the women, were addicted to it. Later, the coffee- and chocolate-loving libertine the Marquis de Sade did much to bolster chocolate's long-rumored (but unproven) reputation for aphrodisiac qualities.

Another indication of chocolate's lofty reputation in Europe was the name bestowed upon it by Carl Linnaeus, the eighteenth-century Swedish botanist who developed the binomial system for identifying species. His name for the tree was *Theobroma cacao*. The latter came from the Mayan word for the tree; the former, taken from Greek, means "food of the gods." (Theobromine, an alkaloid very similar to caffeine, later took its name from the tree; it is far more abundant in chocolate than in caffeine, but it has minimal stimulant effects.)

⚡

Sure, chocolate tastes great. But "food of the gods"? A beverage to drink in concert with human sacrifice? A commodity so valuable that it stood in lieu of gold for money? It is hard to imagine exactly what caused this chocolate lust . . . unless we think about the caffeine.

These days, we don't consider chocolate as a primary source of caffeine, but it would have been a big part of the attraction for the Izapans, and even the pre-coffee Spaniards.

We can't know exactly how much caffeine was contained in the historic cacao drinks, but an analysis of modern chocolate gives some perspective. A Scharffen Berger 82 percent cacao extra-dark chocolate bar has forty-two milligrams of caffeine per forty-three-gram serving (the same size as a standard Hershey bar). That equals roughly a milligram of caffeine per gram of chocolate. If the Izapans made drinks with seventy-five grams of cacao, they would have delivered about a SCAD, the kick of a Red Bull or a single shot of espresso. For anyone not habituated to daily caffeine use, that is a good, solid bump.

One of the reasons we no longer think of chocolate as a primary source of caffeine is that it has been so dramatically adulterated and diluted. A Hershey's milk chocolate bar—forty-three grams—has but nine milligrams of caffeine. Hershey, like most mass-market chocolate makers, skates close to the edge of FDA regulations, which require that milk chocolate include a minimum of 10 percent chocolate liquor. (On nomenclature: Cacao, or chocolate liquor, is the pure product of the bean; cocoa is the dried, processed cacao, with the fatty cocoa butter removed; chocolate is the product we commonly consume, which can range from strong dark chocolate to dilute milk chocolate.)

To understand why chugging down a cold, frothy, unsweetened cacao drink might have appealed to an Izapan ruler (chocolate was then scarce enough that the plebes could not imbibe), it is helpful to understand what happens when we drink caffeinated beverages, whether they're made from cacao or coffee or tea:

Set your stopwatch. Once the liquid hits your stomach, you have about twenty minutes until that gentle buzz hits your brain. Caffeine is unusually mobile in the body. A small molecule, it easily hurdles the blood-brain barrier. In the synaptic stew of our crania, the molecule blocks the uptake of a neurotransmitter called adenosine (pronounced uh-DEN-uh-seen). Adenosine tells the brain we are drowsy, but caffeine does not let the brain get the message. It is this simple trick, elbowing adenosine off the barstool and sitting in its place, that makes caffeine America's favorite drug.

And it is not just hitting your brain. Caffeine has a number of significant, but sometimes contradictory, effects on your physiology. It stimulates your central nervous system. Your alertness increases, your reaction time decreases, and your focus sharpens. Your blood pressure will increase slightly. Your heart may race (but may, in habitual users, actually slow). And in your brain, despite your increased acuity, blood flow will decrease. (It is the inverse of this, the increased blood flow to expanding capillaries, that gives so many caffeine junkies the pounding withdrawal headaches we so dread.)

Once the caffeine locks in on those adenosine receptors, things look rosy; no is task insurmountable. Breaths come easily and deep. You feel so good, how about one more shot of that magical elixir?

Or not. That "sweet spot," the zone where physical and mental performance is optimal, is not wide, and it is easy to blast right on past. Caffeine researcher Scott Killgore told me that caffeine does more than just block adenosine. It has a variety of effects on the mind and body. "At higher doses it can lead to alterations in your heart rhythm. So you can start to have increased heart rate, or tachycardia. . . . So you start to notice that your heart feels like it's pounding very hard or very quickly or maybe skips a beat. And that's a clear indication that you are probably taking too much caffeine in your diet and you need to slow down," he said.

Another clue to excessive caffeine use is a bad mood. "It can make you irritable," said Killgore, "make you more likely to respond in an irritable way to people." Confusing matters, irritability can also be a symptom of caffeine withdrawal.

But these days it is hard to take too much caffeine from chocolate. Because it's become so diluted and other caffeine delivery mechanisms so much more popular, a recent analysis showed that chocolate accounts for just 2.3 milligrams of Americans' daily caffeine consumption (about 1 percent of our total caffeine intake).

⚡

In the Izapan era, cacao was the only caffeine in town. The hot, wet region was perfect for its cultivation. The demand for cacao was so great that historians surmise it was the reason for Izapa's wealth. Today's Izapan cacao groves are not farms in the traditional Western sense. They are managed agroforestry ecosystems bearing multiple crops—from the tall avocado and mamey trees in the canopy down to the cacao growing in the shade near the forest floor. It is an ancient form of agriculture, and one that is now under siege.

Early one bright, fresh morning in Tapachula, I met Rubiel Velasquez Toledo at Red Maya CASFA, an organic growers' cooperative. We were heading out for a tour of cacao country.

I had eaten a light breakfast at the hotel—fresh rolls, a fruit salad made with local mango, papaya, pineapple, and banana, and a couple of cups of café con leche. But out on the highway, Velasquez suggested a bit more sustenance and a taste of local cacao culture.

He pulled his battered Ford pickup over at a roadside stand with a clean cement floor, metal roof, and open sides. Two women stood at the ready, selling the cacao-based drink pozol.

Pozol is an ancient blend, a mixture of cacao and fermented, coarsely ground corn. To prep the drinks, the women rolled the corn and cacao into balls a bit smaller than a baseball. They placed these into a cup with water, used a broad wooden spoon to vigorously blend it, added a dipper of viscous cane sugar, then added ice.

About the color of a chocolate milk shake, pozol has a thick, rich texture, the cacao velvety on the tongue. Velasquez said the hearty drinks are popular with laborers, because the sustenance from the corn and cacao combined with the kick from the caffeine ensures that you don't have to eat again until evening. All of this for eight pesos—about sixty cents.

This is not the only cacao-and-corn drink in the region. Janine Gasco, a California anthropologist and an expert on Soconusco cacao culture, gave me some background before my travels and told me I should also look for tascalate. After some searching, I found it on the menu of a café just off Tapachula's zocalo, or main square. It is a delicious blend of cacao and toasted corn, colored red with the local dye achiote, and served cold. Tascalate feels granular on the tongue, with a bit of a corn tortilla flavor. This might evoke an image of a tortilla chip dipped in milk chocolate, but it tastes nothing like that—both the cacao and the corn are subtle, combining for a rich flavor.

With the exception of the sugar, an innovation that came with the European conquest, these drinks are similar to the frothy chocolate so beloved by the Izapans, the Mayans, and the Aztecs.

$$\nLightning$$

From the pozol stand, Velasquez took me rattling down a dirt road between farms near the town of Plan de Ayala. The villages featured thatched-roof huts, chickens, mules, and scrawny dogs sniffing out a living at the dusty roadside.

Velasquez pulled his truck over to point out a traditional cacao grove. It is the sort of tropical forest we can all easily imagine—verdant, full of exotic birdcalls, with all manner of strange reptiles likely hidden in the dank shadows of the understory. Cedar, oak, avocado, and mango trees grew high above, shading the cacao growing below.

Cacao is a small tree. But it is easy to pick out, even for this amateur naturalist, because its fruits are distinctive—the green, football-shaped pods grow straight out from the trunk. They look like trees Dr. Seuss might have sketched.

Velasquez said this is the traditional, age-old style of cacao farming, in diversified woods with crops at multiple levels. Each layer of the forest produces a cash or food crop—fruit, firewood, or chocolate. But then he pointed to the other side of the road, where a massive field was completely denuded of trees. A new crop of sugarcane was just coming up through the raw dirt. Up until last year, Velasquez said, this was a cacao plantation. Back in the truck, we saw the same story at farm after farm; mile after mile of formerly forested cacao groves had been cleared for not just oil palm and sugarcane but also grains like soy and fruits like papaya. These are massive monocultures, typically owned by foreign agro-biz giants. Once cleared, the land is so raw that even here, with a hundred inches of rain annually, it must be irrigated.

It was siesta time when Velasquez and I reached the last stop on our tour of Chiapas cacao country: Chocolates Finos San José, a small-ish operation on a tidy lot.

Velasquez pulled the truck in, but we saw nobody about. He went to the house while I waited in the shade of a thatched-roof pavilion, where a slight breeze made the heat bearable. Roosters crowed in the distance, turkeys clucked, a listless dog lay in the dust, and a shirtless man in khakis and a rope belt snoozed in a hammock ten feet away, his jellies kicked off. I heard the faint strains of a Mexican ballad playing from a nearby house, the chorus a mournful cry answered by a blast of horns.

Velasquez soon returned from the house with Bernardina Cruz, the diminutive *dueña*. She looked tired. It turned out she had made a batch of chocolate the night before, a process she can't start until nearly midnight, when the heat subsides (the chocolate melts at about ninety degrees). In fact, this is one of the secrets to chocolate's enduring appeal—it is solid at room temperature but melts quickly over the tongue.

Cruz opened the door to her chocolate factory. It was not until we walked in and I smelled the rich chocolate and began to salivate that I realized I had not eaten anything, nor been a bit hungry, since we had the pozol more than seven hours earlier.

The factory is small: a barrel roaster in one room, a milling machine and a refiner in another. Cruz hand-pours the finished chocolate into molds. It is chocolate production on a human scale. She makes about twenty cases of twenty-four chocolate bars daily, processing four tons a year. Some of the chocolate bars are exported to Italy, some go to Germany, and some stay in Mexico and are sold in Guadalajara. At a table next to her small glass-front cooler—like a two-door soda refrigerator at a corner store—she gave me samples of her nibs and chocolate.

Nibs are pieces of roasted chocolate a bit bigger than coarsely ground coffee. Fairly stable in this form, nibs are often shipped as raw ingredients. And they are delicious. Since the cocoa butter has not yet been squeezed out, the crunchy little cacao shards have a hearty, nutty flavor. (Cocoa butter is the most valuable part of the cacao bean; once it is squeezed from the bean, it is often shunted off for use in cosmetics and pharmaceuticals.)

I could eat the freshly roasted organic cacao nibs all day. It is hard to imagine how chocolate evolved to such an extent that most of us are unfamiliar with these nutty, caffeine-rich nibs, knowing only the pale shadow that is modern milk chocolate.

⚡

For years, some claimed the Soconusco region was more than the birthplace of chocolate culture, that it was also the ancestral home of the cacao plant. But USDA researchers showed genetic evidence that cacao was first domesticated in the Upper Amazon. Their published research went even further, refining cacao into ten genetic groups, all present in the small region that is the epicenter of cacao. In their view, cacao was domesticated in what is now northern Peru and southern

Colombia, likely for its sweet fruit, which was used to make beer (the bean itself was not then the object of desire), and then carried north thousands of years ago to the Soconusco. It does seem clear that the Soconusco is where cacao was first used to make chocolate.

Mars Inc. funded this genetic research. The science is critical to the global chocolate industry. West Africa now produces the vast majority of the world's cacao harvest, which has grown quickly—it totaled 4.73 million tons in 2011. The world's cacao harvest has more than tripled since 1960, with Africa accounting for most of the growth. African nations produce six times as much cacao as all the countries in the Americas combined; the Ivory Coast alone produces three times as much. (The African cacao industry owes some of its productivity to child labor, and advocates have prodded Hershey and Nestlé to more effectively fight the practice.)

Two devastating cacao fungi—frosty pod rot and the witches' broom that recently wiped out Brazil's cacao industry—have not yet reached Africa. But diseases endemic to other African plants have found cacao to be a good host and could someday wreak havoc on New World crops. Meanwhile, frosty pod rot has reached Chiapas, further threatening the historic cacao groves near Izapa.

⚡

The evening after touring cacao country with Velasquez, I was cooling my heels at the International Fair of Tapachula. Sipping a coffee granita, a pound of local chocolate in my backpack, I finally had time to read the paper. The lead story was the Chiapas governor's effort to prop up an eco-friendly business. Cacao, you might think? No, palm oil, produced from plantations of nonnative African oil palms to be exported for biodiesel. Ironically, the Chiapas oil palm displacing the cacao groves is being grown with government support to meet the demand of green-leaning consumers in more prosperous countries.

The environmental benefits of preserving cacao groves are now attracting the interest of conservationists like Edward Millard, who oversees sustainable landscapes for the Rainforest Alliance. Millard works from London, but when I finally pinned him down to talk on the phone, he was at a meeting in Costa Rica. He said the alliance is interested in cacao because it is grown on more than seventeen million acres of land that is important for biodiversity. He said over the past twenty years there has been a move to intensify cacao production at the expense of the environment in places like the Ivory Coast, but he believes there is a trend swinging back toward traditional methods, which he welcomes.

"If you can produce a major cash crop like cacao in an understory with a mix of other crops in the same farming system, and all of them together giving you a system to keep your climate healthy, your soils regulated, giving you compost material, et cetera, that's a pretty viable system," said Millard. To support this practice, the Rainforest Alliance is now certifying chocolate that is sustainably harvested.

⚡

Before I left Chiapas, I went back to the Tapachula co-op to see Jorge Aguilar Reyna, its executive director. His office was back in a rabbit warren of rooms opening onto a courtyard. Wooden planks made a walkway over the mud, and a thatched-roof structure with open sides that served as a meeting room housed a long table. Above the table were a large map of the cacao-producing areas, results of cacao taste tests pinned to a sheet of plywood, and a painting of the Virgin Mary.

Aguilar told me he wants to see Americans buying not just Soconusco chocolate, but any chocolate that has a high percentage of cacao. Much of the finished chocolate from the Soconusco region has 30 to 70 percent cacao, far more than popular American milk chocolate bars. And to replace the displaced cocoa butter, the biggest chocolate companies use a castor oil–based emulsifier known as PGPR. Aguilar said it is all part of a "culture of adulteration" that is bad for consumers . . . and bad for cacao farmers.

Aguilar's concerns hit close to home. Even along this Pacific Coast of Mesoamerica, the cradle of chocolate culture, the top-shelf candy bars in the stores are made by Hershey.

Leaving Aguilar's office, I noticed two plastic bags on the corner of his desk: One held green coffee beans; the other was full of dried, unroasted cacao. Unable to resist, I asked if the cacao could be eaten just like that. Sure, he said. He popped one of the cacao beans into his mouth and passed the bag to me. I grabbed one, chewed it, and found its flavor both slightly nutty and bitter, and delicious.

It is not only the oldest known caffeine tradition, but Soconusco chocolate also exemplifies trends that extend across caffeinated products, from tea to coffee to caffeine powder. Two tracks are diverging. On one, the gourmet, artisanal, single-source products are getting more attention from foodies and conservation-minded consumers. On the other, mass-market caffeine delivery mechanisms are going gangbusters. The latter track, no surprise, is where the volume is, even if the former is seeing rapid growth.

As artisanal, single-origin chocolate becomes more popular, the Soconusco is attracting more attention from American chocolatiers. Askinosie Chocolate, in Missouri, has produced limited runs of chocolate bars from pure Soconusco cacao, as has Taza Chocolate, in Massachusetts. Cacao-rich dark chocolate bars not only have significantly more caffeine than commercial milk chocolate; they are also bursting with the health-lending antioxidants known as flavonols.

Raw food advocates are even getting into cacao beans, which are developing a reputation as a superfood. Or have developed that reputation, I should say. The tenacious German explorer Alexander von Humboldt, who traveled the Americas extensively in the early 1800s (and wrote many volumes about his discoveries), summed it up well: "The cocoa bean is a phenomenon, for nowhere else has nature concentrated such a wealth of valuable nourishment in so small a space."

As Americans have gravitated toward darker gourmet chocolate bars, Hershey has gotten a piece of the action. It bought two West Coast chocolate makers—Scharffen Berger and Dagoba—shut down their plants, and centralized production in the Midwest (the bars still look homegrown, funky, and noncorporate, and the labels do not mention Hershey). Unlike the familiar Hershey's bars, these do deliver a caffeine kick.

Though its caffeine has often gotten short shrift, chocolate has long had appeal as a metabolically altering substance. In her book about Hershey and Mars, Joël Glenn Brenner writes, "We still speak of chocolate as if speaking of a drug. It is addicting, sinful, wickedly rich. We crave it, overdose on it and suffer from chocolate withdrawal. A 'fix' of chocolate can relieve depression and calm anxiety. It provides strength and stamina—the perfect pick-me-up between meals."

Brenner could be describing my roadside pozol. And long before the word *chocoholics* came into vogue, chocolate lovers described the habit, and its stimulating qualities, in terms that sound more familiar to coffee drinkers today.

Thomas Gage, the intrepid runaway missionary who traveled through Mexico and Guatemala in the 1600s, wrote detailed accounts of chocolate preparation in his book *Travels in the New World*. It is also interesting to read his account of his own chocolate use: "For myself I must say I used it twelve years constantly, drinking one cup in the morning, another yet before dinner between nine or ten of the clock, another within an hour or after dinner, and another between four and five in the afternoon, and when I was purposed to sit up late to study, I would take another cup about seven or eight at night, which would keep me waking till about midnight."

Gage wrote this more than a century before the word *caffeine* came into use, but clearly he already knew of its stimulating powers. And the Chinese, thousands of miles across the Pacific, were way ahead of him.

CHAPTER 2

All the Tea in China

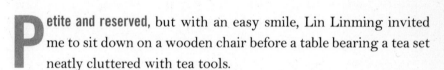

Petite and reserved, but with an easy smile, Lin Linming invited me to sit down on a wooden chair before a table bearing a tea set neatly cluttered with tea tools.

She used a wooden scoop to fetch some tea from a wicker bin. It was a puer tea, which is an aged tea harvested in 2006 in China's Yunnan province. The tray before her, carved of dark wood, is called "the sea of tea." At the far end is a carved "tea pet," a figurine that looks like a toad with a smiling Buddha face. Lin's tea pet is called the Nice Son of the Dragon God.

She heated water in an electric kettle on a low shelf behind her. She poured some into a teapot, of course, but also, ritualistically, into a small bowl full of tea leaves, over the tea pet and the sea of tea, and onto some peanuts as an offering. Then Lin poured tea for me and my companions: my translator, Aida Leng, and Xie Yanchen, a tea expert and editor at *Beijing Youth Daily*.

The whole process was imbued with ritual, much of it ancient, as tea drinking has evolved in Asia over thousands of years. If the Soconusco can claim the earliest documented use of caffeine, the Chinese can claim the earliest use by folkloric tradition: five thousand years ago.

By this account, the emperor Shennong was boiling water to drink when some tea leaves blew into the pot. He drank the brew, noticed its stimulating effects, and thus gave birth to tea culture. It is notable that the tale does not credit tea's flavor or calming properties for opening the emperor's eyes to the plant's possibilities, but its caffeine kick. (Shennong was a productive herbalist with a keen eye for medicine; he is also credited with discovering ephedra, ginseng, and marijuana.)

To get a sense of just how huge tea culture has become in the intervening centuries, it is helpful to understand the southwest Beijing neighborhood in which Lin's store sits.

The store is on Maliandao Street, a.k.a. Tea Street. This is the world's largest tea market, with more than three thousand tea shops in just a few blocks in Beijing. As you pass by each stall, the shopkeepers beckon you in to taste the wares. If you do step in, it is not for a quick chug. When you enter a tea shop, you are in for a genuine tea experience—no tea bags in tepid water here.

As we sipped our tea, rich with a slightly smoky flavor, Xie explained that tea is more than just China's favorite caffeinated beverage; it is also a key part of daily social life. There are basically three ways to enjoy tea in China. If a friend visits your house, it is a hospitable tradition to offer her some tea. And you might go out with friends for tea, as Americans often do for coffee. Most elaborately, there are the exclusive teahouses with highly ritualized programs featuring traditional Chinese music and art, performance, and Zen philosophy.

Lin poured more water from the teakettle onto the leaves, then she poured more tea all around. To thank her, we subtly tapped our first two fingers twice on the tabletop. (This is known as the "finger kowtow"; the bent digits represent kneeling in gratitude.)

Xie told us that puer is good for the stomach and especially good for women because "puer is warm, and women are cold." During Chinese New Year, when people eat too much, or when eating hot pot (a spicy, greasy style of cooking), they drink puer tea to get rid of toxins. She said it is also good for aging people, because it helps to lower their blood pressure. Traditional Chinese people pay close attention to health, she said, correlating types of teas with different times of the year: In spring, herbal tea helps to get rid of viruses and other sickness and protects the body; green tea is considered cold, helping you cool down in summer; and in autumn and winter, rat or black tea helps to warm you up.

But I was wondering about the caffeine in tea. Its effects have been well-known for decades. In a 1931 essay, Albert G. Nicholls had this to say: "Perhaps we can find the solution for the popularity of tea-drinking in the effect of caffeine on the central nervous system, particularly that part associated with the psychic functions. Cushny, an authority on pharmacology, says—'The ideas become clearer, thought flows more easily and rapidly, and fatigue and drowsiness disappear. . . .' The capacity for physical exertion is augmented, as has been demonstrated repeatedly in the case of soldiers on the march."

So I asked Xie and Lin, what about the caffeine? Although Xie replied, "We don't just use it to wake up," Lin countered that she had recently met some young professionals from Beijing who asked which tea is best as a stimulant.

One American in particular has been asking a version of the caffeine question. Bruce Goldberger could be a character in the HBO series *The Wire*. The forensic toxicologist used to work in Baltimore and was often called on to identify the lethal drug in the blood of overdose victims. When I called him at his office in Gainesville, Florida, he explained his work like this: "Most of my work is in the area of death investigation, medical or legal death investigation—why do people die from drugs?—and assisting medical examiners in the declaration and certification of cause and manner of death."

But Goldberger has also turned his analytical mind to a question with broader appeal: How much caffeine are we getting in our beverages? The project started when he was talking to a friend. "She was

working at a coffee shop in Baltimore, and she would serve these dou-
ble- and triple-shot lattes to customers, and people would come in and
get coffee three or four times a day," Goldberger said. "And that
spurred my interest in wondering how much caffeine are they actually
getting?"

Goldberger first studied the caffeine contents of coffee, then went
on to do a series of studies on other caffeinated products, demystifying
the caffeine kick.

In his 2008 study on tea, Goldberger found that the caffeine content increased with the length of steeping time. So a bag of Lipton tea
steeped for one minute had a mere seventeen milligrams of caffeine;
after three minutes, thirty-eight milligrams; after five, forty-seven
milligrams. Most teas steeped for three minutes had between twenty-
five and fifty milligrams of caffeine, about half a SCAD. Surprisingly,
Goldberger's finding bucked the popular notion that green teas are
always less caffeinated than black teas. Tazo China Green Tips tea had
more caffeine than Twinings Earl Grey or English Breakfast teas.

Goldberger and his colleagues noted that Lipton was alone, among
the teas they analyzed, in listing milligrams of caffeine per serving.
"Lipton reports concentrations of 55 mg/serving for its regular tea
and 5 mg/serving for its decaffeinated tea, which are, in fact, consistent with the findings of this study," they wrote. "Declaring the caffeine content on product labels is important for consumers wishing to
limit caffeine intake."

It may be partly due to the lack of quantified caffeine labels, but as
his caffeine studies stacked up, Goldberger realized that most of us
don't know much about caffeine.

"Based on the questions I've gotten over the last decade, I think
people are pretty naive," he told me. "They know that beverages contain caffeine. But they can't quantify it. The best measuring stick for
them would be NoDoz, which contains two hundred milligrams of
caffeine. And a lot of people would say, 'I would never eat a NoDoz.
That's crazy.' But that wouldn't stop them from drinking two or three

Starbucks coffees a day—that could result in more than a gram of caffeine ingestion. So no, they don't really understand, or can't quantify, the amount of caffeine they take."

This inability to quantify caffeine intake may be the source of what I believe is a misperception. I've heard from some tea drinkers who prefer its mellower effects to the coffee kick, which they call "an angry buzz." This is often attributed to the calming properties of theanine, another chemical constituent of tea.

Theanine does have some effect on mental function. Several recent studies have found that the combination of caffeine and theanine improves mood and alertness more than caffeine alone. At high doses, theanine alone (without caffeine) can even improve alertness among anxious individuals. Clearly, then, theanine is not inert. But in nature, you will only find it alongside caffeine.

Attempting to capitalize on its reputation as a calming substance, which is still unsettled in the scientific literature, a team of Japanese researchers has actually claimed a patent for a method to counter the caffeine buzz with theanine. Their solution is to extract theanine from tea and blend it into coffee to allow caffeine-sensitive people to enjoy the aroma and flavor without getting too jacked up. (Decaffeinated coffee would be a simpler and far more effective solution.)

My suspicion is that the primary distinction between the angry buzz of coffee and the mellower buzz of tea has most to do with the average differences in caffeine content. A six-ounce cup of coffee will often have a SCAD or more, easily twice the amount of a six-ounce cup of tea. It is a consistently stronger buzz, and if that's not what you are after, it's easy to see how that might seem like an angry buzz.

Whatever the quality of the buzz, tea is still a small percentage of Americans' collective caffeine dose. On average, Americans take a mere twenty-four milligrams of caffeine from tea daily, a tenth of our total caffeine consumption. We get nearly twice as much caffeine from soft drinks and six times as much from coffee.

Whenever we discuss our tea habits, the conversation invariably turns to British tea drinking. By legend, Americans' affinity for coffee and aversion to tea were rooted in patriotism, vestiges of the country-catalyzing Boston Tea Party. It is a convenient myth, but only partly true. Coffee also appealed to Americans in this country's early years because it was closer at hand—much of it produced by slave labor in Haiti—and easier to procure without running afoul of British traders.

Anyone will tell you that the British have remained allied with tea, not coffee. But that, too, is only partly true. While the British drink more tea, by volume, than coffee, they now get more of their caffeine from coffee than from tea. Surprisingly, colas and energy drinks now contribute nearly as much caffeine to the British diet as tea: thirty-four milligrams daily versus thirty-six milligrams daily.

⚡

From Lin's shop, we went across the street to Ya Xiang Tea, where Yang Shuhan invited us to sit for a tasting. She poured us Iron Buddha, an oolong tea with a distinctive, floral aroma.

All true tea (distinct from herbal tea) comes from the same plant, *Camellia sinensis*. This one tea plant can produce green or black tea, depending on how it is processed. Green tea is made from the unfermented tea leaves, black tea from the fermented tea leaves, and oolong tea from partially fermented leaves.

Next, we tasted a black tea, Jing Jun Mei. A fully fermented tea, it smells rich and funky, like sweet potatoes. Then we tried a roasted oolong from 2005 called Da Hong Pao, or Big Red Robe. These teas are roasted again every year to refresh the leaves. After she poured the tea into a clear glass beaker, Yang held it up to the light and showed us tiny feathery particles just barely visible in the water, a mark of quality.

She and Xie began conversing rapidly in Chinese about different varieties of tea and the origin stories that accompany their colorful names. All of the fine teas we tasted were dried into what looked like loose little pellets, not the leaves or leaf fragments usually sold as loose teas in the United States. But add water and an entire tea leaf unfurls. Xie shared something she had written in one of her books on tea: Our lives are like tea leaves; they expand and transform over time.

We talked briefly about bottled, ready-to-drink teas. Xie said she would not buy them. Yang agreed. She said, "They are made from leftovers and have artificial additives." These additives often include sweeteners, potassium sorbate, and other preservatives that make some bottled teas seem more like flat soft drinks than iced tea.

They said that large Western tea companies also use leftover tea leaves and powder. It is true that most American tea companies use tea that would be considered substandard in China or India, because it includes shredded pieces of tea leaves instead of the entire leaf. Since the teas will most often be brewed in bags, smaller pieces are fine for many Western tea traders. This does not necessarily mean the tea has inferior flavor.

"Tea bags are very casual, convenient, but real tea lovers do not think they are very good," Xie said. "This is a fast-food lifestyle, but Chinese people like whole foods."

I later talked to Eugene Amici, an American tea importer, and he outlined the contrasting tea cultures in a nutshell. "Here, you put a dollar into a machine, you pop the top and drink it, and you roll," he said. "For them, it's an afternoon."

Amici said the vast majority of the tea consumed in this country is not taken as we commonly think of it, as a tea bag in a teacup, steeping in hot water. About 85 percent is used for iced tea. This might be bottled or the pitchers of "sweet tea" that lubricate southern restaurant dining (these are often brewed from tea bags, but the bags are the size of laptop computers and make four gallons of tea).

According to the Tea Association of the USA, tea consumption is growing steadily. In 2011, the United States imported more tea than the United Kingdom. Much of that growth is in ready-to-drink bottled teas (or RTD, in the industry jargon).

Ready-to-drink tea sales increased seventeen-fold between 2001 and 2011; sales exceeded $3.5 billion in 2011.

The bottled tea business began growing just as sales of carbonated soft drinks started to slowly decline from their 1998 peak. Much of this growth likely comes from people switching over from soft drinks, due to the perception that bottled teas are healthier. But some of the bottled teas actually pack in more sugar than Coke, which seems like it would quickly offset any benefit from the diluted tea in the blend. Anyway, bottled teas have quickly become an extension of the global soft drink industry.

As soft drinks peaked in 1998, Seth Goldman founded Honest Tea to market organic bottled teas (he calls himself the TeaEO). The company has grown like wildfire—so much that Coca-Cola took notice and bought the company in 2011.

In 2008, Starbucks partnered with Pepsi and Unilever to bottle, market, and distribute a line of bottled teas under the Tazo brand (which Starbucks bought in 1999). Pepsi and Unilever were already involved in a joint venture to produce bottled teas under the Pepsi Lipton Tea Partnership, which is atop the heap in the bottled tea sector.

While these mass-market tea products are going gangbusters, the specialty, or gourmet, tea sector is also thriving. As just one indicator of its promise, Sara Lee in 2012 acquired Tea Forté, a high-end Massachusetts company. In a press release, Sara Lee called the products "ultrapremium" and "luxury" teas. It may seem incongruous to serve gourmet tea in bags, but they are not bags, according to Tea Forté—they are "pyramid infusers." The company markets tea as "the healthiest beverage on earth."

It is these changes—the bottled teas, the jugs of sweet tea, and the gourmet teas—that infuse the American tea market with its current vigor. The new products have allowed tea to cling to its small but significant share of America's caffeine dose. It is still tea, and it is still caffeinated, although it seems a long way from Maliandao Street. But really it's not.

Leaving Maliandao in the twilit, gridlocked rush hour, we passed a tiny corner store, open to the street. It was selling bottled Lipton tea, bottled Coke, canned coffee, and Red Bull. In the back of the cluttered stall was a TV showing a recent Red Bull parachute stunt. Was it an ad that just happened to be on as we passed or a looping video? I did not linger long enough to find out.

CHAPTER 3

High on the Mountain

At the southern edge of the Caribbean Sea, in northern Colombia, rises a mighty mountain range, the Sierra Nevada de Santa Marta. Its glacier-capped summits reach nearly nineteen thousand feet, set back just twenty-five miles from the sandy beaches. To grasp its topographic extravagance, picture Denali rising behind the Art Deco hotels of South Beach.

They are mountains that do many things well—growing marijuana and coca, hosting strange and colorful wildlife, and hiding fugitives. Descending from the snowfields toward the coast, there are high-altitude plains, then the humid cloud forests, which are home to dozens of native birds and frogs. Here, too, are the remote reserves of the indigenous tribes, austere people descended from the ancient Tayrona civilization.

Farther downslope in remote folds of the mountains are more than a thousand acres of clandestine coca patches tended by the feuding outlaws who also share this space—leftist guerrillas and murderous paramilitary blocs. Before cocaine became so popular, the area was famous for the potent pot known as Santa Marta Gold. But weed and cocaine are not the only drugs grown here.

Standing on a hillside path above a rutted dirt road, farmer David Castilla showed me a handful of beans cupped in his callused palm. Each pale yellow bean was the size of a small peanut. The mid-elevation zone has just the right blend of moderate precipitation and strong tropical sunshine for the beans to grow abundantly on small-ish, glossy-leafed trees.

Like coca leaves, the beans are laden with a psychoactive alkaloid compound, a simple blend of carbon, hydrogen, nitrogen, and oxygen that is easily refined to a bitter white powder. Castilla was holding coffee beans, packed with caffeine, the world's most popular drug.

If not for the caffeine, coffee would still be just a shrub growing in the hills of North Africa, where, as the apocryphal tale has it, goats nibbled on the plant and suddenly started dancing. Intrigued, a goat herder sampled the beans and started feeling frisky himself, singing and reciting poetry. For hundreds of years coffee was used in its raw form—astringent and bitter—boiled or rolled with animal fat into a crude approximation of energy pellets. People clearly were chomping the coffee berries for the buzz, not the flavor. Yes, modern coffee tastes great. But it is four hundred years of selective breeding and refine-ments in growing, harvesting, roasting, and brewing that have taken it from its unappealing natural state to the aromatic, smooth, flavorful beverage it has become. And without the caffeine, nobody would have bothered with the plant in the first place.

The association between coffee and caffeine is historic. Caffeine was first refined by the German scientist Friedlieb Runge, at the behest of his friend Johann Wolfgang von Goethe. Runge extracted the caffeine from coffee. This association is so important that the English-language word *caffeine* is derived from the German word for coffee: *Kaffee*. And the association continues today. Among all Americans, about two-thirds of our caffeine consumption (more than one hundred milli-grams daily, a bit more than a SCAD) comes from coffee. And those of us who drink coffee daily skew the statistics, because we take far more caffeine than other Americans, a bit more than three hundred milligrams daily, or four SCADs. Any way you slice the statistics, coffee is far and away the largest source of caffeine for Americans, and it is easy to see why many people think of coffee and caffeine interchangeably.

⚡

David Castilla gave me a tour of his coffee farm, where dozens of glossy-leafed, evergreen coffee trees, eight to fifteen feet tall, were growing in partial shade. Some of the trees had berries growing along their branches. The size and color of a cranberry when ripe, the fleshy berries envelop the seed that is the coffee bean.

This is arabica coffee, the species native to the mountains of Ethiopia, where it evolved with a blend of drenching rains, abundant sun, and a narrow band of acceptable temperature. Arabica is the smooth-flavored coffee Americans have come to love, the coffee that gourmet coffee connoisseurs swear by. The other common commercially grown coffee species is robusta, which is heartier and more productive and can grow in warmer temperatures, out in the open at low elevation. Robusta beans are often blended into commercial coffees, like Folgers. But virtually all Colombian coffee is arabica.

After a brief tour of the coffee farm, I sat with a small group on the cement patio where Castilla dries his coffee beans in the sun, next to his small house.

Castilla pulled out a battered can filled with coffee he'd roasted on his wood-fired cookstove, poured a handful into the funnel atop a large hand-cranked grinder clamped to a plank wood table, and ground it to a fine, dark powder before pouring it directly into a pot of water boiling on the cookstove. He served me some of the strong, fresh coffee, nearly brimful in a chipped porcelain cup.

It wasn't great. Most of the best coffee produced in Colombia is sold for export. Like much of the coffee served in rural Colombia, it was made from leftover beans, roasted to blackness, ground nearly to powder, then boiled into sludge. You could get a better cup at any Dunkin' Donuts or 7-Eleven, not to mention Starbucks or Stumptown.

But it was also one of the most memorable cups of coffee of my life. It felt fantastic to sip coffee on the farm where the beans were grown, roasted, and ground, listening to the woods full of birdsong, watching huge hummingbirds hover over flowering vines next to the patio, looking down over the mango trees to see turkey vultures soaring above the hills rolling out toward the Caribbean.

Then I caught a glimpse of something faint in the periphery, a motion in the distance, through the trees. Something passing on the road? A distant *click, clomp*? My ears pricked up a bit. We were in an area with a history of conflict between guerrillas and paramilitary troops, and I was feeling a little paranoid.

The motion on the road became more conspicuous and the metallic noise louder. Soon I saw them coming down off the hill—a man and a mule. The mule carried a pack frame loaded up with two massive burlap sacks. They passed us, the man giving a benign wave and no hint of menace. Relieved, I couldn't help but think he looked somewhat familiar.

Soon after, it occurred to me why this was. He was reminiscent of a folk icon who rose from coffee's mid-century doldrums and came to its rescue, complete with white hat and handsome steed. But he was not astride the beast; he was leading it. And it was no horse; it was a mule. As you might have guessed by now, this folk hero is Juan Valdez, created in 1960 by the ad firm Doyle Dane Bernbach for the National Federation of Coffee Growers of Colombia.

The alliance between Colombian coffee growers and Madison Avenue admen grew from a desperate situation: a coffee market in crisis. This brings us to something counterintuitive. Despite Americans' conspicuous embrace of gourmet coffee (as exemplified by the Starbucks on seemingly every corner), our grandparents drank more coffee than we do. A lot more.

American coffee consumption peaked in the World War II years. Back then, coffee was flat-out winning in the competition against other beverages. Americans drank forty-six gallons annually—nearly twenty pounds of beans per person. Soldiers drank it from large enameled tin cups. Women working in factories, Rosie the Riveter style, guzzled it during their breaks. On the radio, the Ink Spots sang "Java Jive." Frank Sinatra sang, "Way down among Brazilians, coffee beans grow by the billions, so they've got to find those extra cups to fill. They've got an awful lot of coffee in Brazil."

Capitalizing on coffee's peaking popularity, the Pan American Coffee Bureau coined the phrase "coffee break" for a massive ad campaign in 1952. "The bureau gave a name and official sanction to a practice that had begun during the war in defense plants, when time off for coffee gave workers a needed moment of relaxation along with a caffeine jolt," wrote Mark Pendergrast in *Uncommon Grounds*. Soon most American companies had institutionalized the coffee break.

But by the late 1950s, facing competition from Coke and other caffeinated soft drinks, coffee consumption was falling just as production was ramping up, leaving the market glutted and prices plummeting. In Colombia, coffee prices dropped by 50 percent.

A young American journalist wrote a letter from Cali, Colombia, to his editor at the *National Observer* in the summer of 1963, describing the situation: "My figures sent earlier on the price of Colombian coffee on the world market are correct, but not nearly as dramatic as the following: ninety cents a pound in 1954, 39 cents a pound in 1962. As I said, Colombia depends on coffee for 77 percent of its export earnings. Incidentally, Colombia gets another 15 percent of its export earnings from petroleum. That leaves 8 percent as a base to begin 'diversifying' with. Not much, eh? Some good minds are just about at the end of their tether with the problem."

This journalist traveling through South America, at a time when few Americans paid much attention to Colombia at all, was Hunter S. Thompson. He had put his finger on a persistent problem in the coffee business: the cycles of glut and dearth that affect coffee more than most commodities.

At that time, only one in twenty coffee consumers even knew that Colombia was a coffee-growing country; the country of origin was of little consequence to coffee drinkers. Not only did roasters not boast of coffee's country of origin, but they preferred to keep it hidden, in order to have more flexibility to blend coffees.

That's when Juan Valdez trudged into newspapers and onto TV screens. Dressed like a simple but proud coffee grower, he emphasized the care farmers took to produce a high-quality cup of coffee. He showed how farmers picked coffee by hand and dried it in the sun. Valdez taught Americans to appreciate coffees of origin, or single-origin coffees, by emphasizing the difference between just any coffee and Colombian coffee. He became one of the best-known pitchmen of the era, alongside the Marlboro Man and the Pillsbury Doughboy.

The ads worked. Colombian coffee started selling at a premium, paving the way for the Starbucks generation of aficionados, who can name not only their favorite coffee-growing country but also the region, and maybe even the farm, where their beans were harvested.

Valdez revolutionized coffee sales by branding Colombian coffee. But he did something more, too. He established a coffee-sales narrative that has become the staple of the gourmet coffee story line: modest but hardworking farmers in far-off lands, proud to deliver you an exceptional cup of coffee. Often as not this story is accompanied—in magazine ads, in annual reports from Green Mountain Coffee Roasters and Starbucks—by what has become an iconic photo: a callused hand cupping the red berries that will eventually make your coffee.

These are hands like the ones that belong to David Castilla, who had picked some coffee berries for us a half hour earlier. They lay on a wooden table at my side, next to my coffee cup. As the mule passed on the road, Castilla did me the favor of pouring more coffee into my cup. Though the past few days had been exhausting, a solid thrash, I soon felt a gentle surge of energy as the caffeine kicked in—hurdling the blood-brain barrier to perform its synaptic magic—bringing on a boost in confidence, an inquisitive acuity.

I'd hitched a ride to Castilla's in an overcrowded Land Rover with several Thai agronomists touring Colombian coffee farms. A representative of the local coffee cooperative was serving as a tour guide, and two idealistic young federal employees had flown in from Medellín to describe Familias Guardabosques, a Colombian initiative to help farmers grow legitimate crops instead of cocaine.

There on the patio, the Colombians described the Guardabosques program to the Thais, explaining that each family who signed up got one hundred dollars a month—not a windfall but a healthy incentive—for eighteen months in exchange for a pledge not to grow illicit crops. Instead, they are growing other valuable crops, like coffee and cacao. More than sixty thousand families had joined the program. Since the cocaine industry is worth billions annually, this might seem like a drop in the ocean, but coffee, too, is worth tens of billions of dollars a year.

At the industry's base are farms like Castilla's, which produces almost nine hundred pounds of coffee per acre. But this farm is just a corpuscle in a capillary in the global caffeine circulatory system. Colombia produces one billion pounds of coffee annually, bringing more than $2 billion into the country each year and trailing only oil and coal in export value among legal commodities.

Although Colombian coffee is well-known, it comprises a small percentage of the annual worldwide coffee harvest, which now exceeds nineteen billion pounds. That is enough coffee to fill more than a million dump trucks—parked end-to-end, they would reach from Seattle to Boston and back to Los Angeles. The industry is worth more than $70 billion annually.

This massive industry feeds an important, if not indispensable, part of most Americans' lives. To brew our average fix of nearly three cups of coffee daily, America imported 3.5 billion pounds of coffee in 2012, more than any other nation. The coffee Americans drink annually would fill more than six thousand Olympic-size swimming pools.

More than half of the adults in the United States drink coffee every

day. It is hard to know which is stranger: that most Americans probably can't remember the last day we skipped coffee or the fact that we
consider this entirely normal.

Once, in a bar, I asked an acquaintance about her coffee habit. She
said coffee is not a big deal to her; she just takes two cups in the morning. So I asked when was the last time she had gone without those two
cups. She paused, thought for a minute, took a sip of beer, and said, "I
guess about thirty-five years."

We are not alone in our love for coffee. In every corner of the globe,
people enjoy coffee in their own specific ways. In Colombia, tinto
(TEEN-toe)—a short cup of black coffee sweetened with cane sugar—is
a constant presence, a social lubricant, especially in rural areas. Run
into an old friend and the first words are, "*Tomamos un tinto.*" Let's
have a coffee. Brazilians, especially the emerging urban middle class,
prefer the short, strong coffee known as cafezinho. Throughout Latin
America, many start their day with a large mug of café con leche: half
coffee, half milk.

In Italy, they take espresso, in small shots, standing at the bar. They
charge a table fee to anyone who wants to sit, so there you stand, an
elbow on the bar, one eye on the barista, the other on the busy street
out the door, having a moment with your coffee. Germans have a similar custom of stand-up coffee at coffeehouses called *Stehcafés*. It's a
brief, pleasant ritual, repeated several times daily. Just don't ask for a
to-go cup.

In Spain, a short, strong cup of espresso with a drop of milk is
called a cortado, meaning it is cut by the milk. Cubans, too, have adopted this habit. Cuban exiles brought it to Miami, where in older
parts of the city you can still buy their cortaditos, often in small Sty-
rofoam cups. The same pattern holds in Puerto Rico, where dignified
old men in guayaberas converse over their cortados in pigeon-filled
parks.

Scandinavians like their coffee strong and abundant. Residents of
Sweden, Norway, Switzerland, and Finland all drink twice as much

coffee as Americans. The average Swede drinks 1,460 cups of coffee annually. This helps to explain the hundred references to coffee in Stieg Larsson's bestseller *The Girl with the Dragon Tattoo*.

Vietnamese prefer robusta coffees, which have nearly twice as much caffeine as the fine, shade-grown arabica that Americans prefer. The two species of coffee are closely related, but robustas are bitter, giving the coffee a tang, which is mellowed by serving it with condensed milk. Thai coffee is the same.

In China, coffee, if you can find it, usually means soluble coffee, a.k.a. instant coffee. It's usually made from robusta beans and typically comes in three-in-one tubes, with powdered creamer and sugar already in place to mask the bitterness.

Japan is the outlier in Asia, having embraced coffee fully. The Japanese have a penchant for low-acid arabicas, especially the mild Colombian coffees. They import these fine coffees, brew them in large vats, and package them in cans, served cold in summer, warm in winter. Coca-Cola sells more than $1 billion worth of Georgia-brand canned coffee annually in Japan. Nescafé Santa Marta au Lait is another popular canned coffee, and Japan accounts for half of the Santa Marta region's coffee exports. So keen are the Japanese on their fine Colombian coffee that a Japanese corporation owns several organic coffee plantations on the Sierra Nevada de Santa Marta, to the west of Castilla's farm.

As we sipped our coffee, Castilla stood in the sunshine on the patio and recited a poem, entreating his neighbors who had abandoned farms for the city to return: "Pretty are our farms with their inherited flowers, and the birds that are happy at five in the morning," it began. As he spoke, with great timing and restrained dramatic flair, another pair of mules laden with produce passed by, headed for town.

We soon piled back into the Land Rover and bounced down the road behind the mules, following the path Castilla's coffee beans take to the narrow coastal plain where the city of Santa Marta perches at the edge of the Caribbean Sea.

On the way back into town, we visited a hotel run by a family that had grown coca but went legit. Fabio Ramirez, one of the owners, offered me a tinto, but then suggested that the gringo might prefer a Coke.

⚡

The next day, wandering through the chaotic, noisy, odiferous streets of Santa Marta, I stumbled onto a Juan Valdez Café in a tree-shaded courtyard. A cool, tranquil eddy in the city bustle. The coffee was fantastic—medium roast, drip filtered, and made from premium beans.

Juan Valdez Cafés are like modern American espresso bars, run by the National Federation of Coffee Growers of Colombia. While Colombians taught Americans to appreciate coffees of origin, Americans provided the Seattle-style template for these coffee bars.

But the international cultural exchange dates back centuries. Coffeehouses first emerged in Mecca, then spread through the Arab world. By the 1600s, they had reached Italy and continued west. Before switching its allegiance to tea, England took quickly to coffee culture; one coffeehouse frequented by sailors and merchants eventually evolved into the famous insurance broker Lloyd's of London. And as coffee culture took root in the American colonies, the insurgents who planned the Boston Tea Party drafted their plans at the coffeehouse/bar known as the Green Dragon Tavern. (Coffee might still fan the revolutionary flame—at Juan Valdez, a stylish young man with long curly hair sat down at the next table, wearing a Che Guevara T-shirt reading "*Hasta la Victoria Siempre.*")

The European coffeehouses morphed into the Parisian cafés haunted by expats and the postwar Italian espresso cafés. Italian émigré Giovanni Giotta brought the espresso café to San Francisco's North Beach, where the beat poets frequented his Caffe Trieste. On the East Coast, the raggedy-shaggedy beat/hippie coffee shops of Greenwich Village gave the coffeehouse movement a bit more literary cachet.

And then along came Starbucks CEO Howard Schultz when, you might say, the cultural pump had been primed for café culture. His

Starbucks bio puts it this way: "In 1983, Howard traveled to Italy and was captivated by Italian coffee bars and the romance of the coffee experience. He had a vision to bring the Italian coffeehouse tradition back to Seattle, creating a third place between work and home."

Schultz understood the allure of the café. That's why Starbucks cafés—even those marooned in the asphalt seas of shopping mall parking lots—feel different than, say, Dunkin' Donuts or McDonald's. It is a matter of softer lighting and fewer plastic surfaces, more jazzy music playing subtly, more armchairs, and especially the aromas of coffee grinding and brewing. Schultz refined the café experience to its elements.

This is the second thing we talk about when we talk about coffee: café culture. The tranquil places to stop for a cup of coffee and have a brief moment to recharge.

From the café, I wandered the two blocks to the shore. Looking out over the harbor in Santa Marta, beyond the fishermen's boats, I saw huge ships loading up at the container port. Some were hauling Dole bananas from nearby plantations. The fine Santa Marta coffee, too, is loaded up from these docks, in twenty-foot containers holding 250 sixty-kilo burlap bags.

Inside those containers, integrated into all of those beans in all of those burlap sacks, is coffee's active ingredient. There are sixteen thousand milligrams of caffeine per sack, which adds up to sixteen million pounds exported from Colombia every year, a wonder drug smuggled out in the coffee beans.

⚡

A good while later, I wound up in Guatemala City, where more than fifteen hundred coffee growers, exporters, and experts from all over the world had converged for the 2010 World Coffee Conference, an event that takes place every five years. It was quite a scene. Throughout a huge exhibit hall wafted the mingled scents of the world's best coffees, from four continents. It was a coffee lover's dream.

Up at the top of the hall, in the prime real estate near the entrance, slender brunettes in bright yellow, skintight, bell-bottom jumpsuits were handing out gift bags stuffed with Mexican coffee, brochures, and travel mugs emblazoned with the Café de Mexico logo. Their four-pump espresso station was doing yeoman's work. Nearby, baristas at the Guatemalan coffee exporters' display were pulling espressos for all comers. The crowd was three deep.

Down at the other end of the room, Ric Rhinehart was sipping coffee and talking to the Panamanian grower Francisco Serracin. Rhinehart, a jovial man with a mustache and jazz patch, is the executive director of the Specialty Coffee Association of America. He knew not only the varieties of trees on Serracin's farm but also their lineages, as a horse trader knows a stallion's parents.

Throughout the hall, coffee traders compared notes, exchanged business cards, renewed old friendships, and told tales of expeditions to coffee farms on far corners of the planet (a.k.a. "going to source"). The caffeine-reinforced cheer was well warranted. Coffee prices had recovered following a glut, and demand was growing quickly, especially in developing countries. In a way, the hall mirrored American cities, where gourmet coffee is better, cheaper, and more available than ever; where once-esoteric terms like *espresso, latte, machiatto*, and *mocha* have become mainstream. The gourmet coffee revolution had actually managed to slightly increase American coffee consumption, about 20 percent since 1995, after the steady decline since the 1950s.

People came to the conference from forty-six countries. Indicating coffee's key economic value in Central America, presidents from three different countries were in attendance: Guatemalan president Alvaro Colom, naturally, and Salvadoran president Mauricio Funes. Also attending, looking cheery, was Porfirio Lobo, the Honduran president, a confident public speaker with a telegenic smile who can deliver a real stem-winder. Lobo had recently assumed power after his predecessor was abducted in a military coup and flown out of the country in his pajamas. If Lobo's situation appeared tenuous, so was Colom's. His government had nearly been toppled nine months earlier by a bizarre scandal that had, somewhere in its deep recesses, involved corruption among coffee growers.

The event also attracted aficionados like coffee consultant Mark Overly, who works in Denver for Kaladi Coffee Roasters. Over dinner one night he explained coffee flavor as a logical sequence of three variables—strength, taste, and aroma—that even an unsophisticated palate can discern. Strength is the body, the viscosity of the coffee in the mouth. Taste can be sweet, salty, sour, or bitter. And then, most complex of all, is the aroma, which can have dozens of permutations.

To help people understand what they are tasting and smelling, Overly uses a coffee wheel that has become the industry standard. It displays a coffee aroma spectrum, running along a continuum of light roast (fruity, herby, flowery) to medium roast (nutty, caramelly, chocolaty) and dark roast (spicy, carbony, resinous). For those who want to delve further, it's got each of the aromas broken down into two more specific categories. "Nutty," for example, can be malt-like or nut-like, and nut-like can give you almond or peanut flavors.

I prefer the soft, neutral flavors often associated with low-acid coffees (coffee blenders like these coffees, too, because they are inoffensive to most people). But many people consider these to be bland at best, boring at worst. Serious coffee connoisseurs often trend toward the bright, fruit-like flavors associated with high acidity.

Where do these strange, complex flavors come from? Typically, they come from well-grown coffee, tended lovingly in fertile soils at high elevations. They come from estates like Finca San Sebastián, in central Guatemala's Antigua Valley, where the volcanic soils, the tropical latitude, and high elevation produce just the right conditions for growing some of the world's best coffee.

The historic city of Antigua is just an hour from traffic-clogged, smoggy, and violent Guatemala City, but with its fresh air, colonial square, and well-preserved buildings, it seems like it exists in an altogether different country. Antigua is dramatically nestled beneath a trio of volcanoes—the Volcán de Acatenango, the Volcán de Agua, and the Volcán de Fuego.

I'd met Estuardo Falla, the fourth-generation manager of Finca San Sebastián, at the conference in Guatemala City and asked if I could come out to see the farm. I arrived ahead of schedule, and Falla, a quietly friendly young man in a peach-colored polo shirt and faded jeans, asked if I wanted to join his other guests, coffee growers and salesmen from Guatemala, Panama, and Colombia, for lunch. We ate in a one-story building with a kitchen behind a wall on one end and a bar two steps up on the other end. Both of the long sides had large windows opening onto the neat grassy fields in the foreground, rows of coffee trees in the middle distance, and the volcanoes rising beyond. With cowhide rugs, rustic leather chairs, tile floors, exposed beams, and a single orchid on the long, wooden dining table, it was the picture of understated elegance and could have been the setting for a Colombian telenovela or a Ralph Lauren ad.

The lunchtime conversation was peppered with talk of some of the common varieties of arabica coffee trees—bourbon, caturra, and typica trees. After lunch we had coffee, of course, brewed in a drip coffeemaker on a sideboard and served as casually as it would be in an American diner. It was as delicious as I expected, with a hint of the tart, citrusy notes that Guatemalan coffee is known for.

From there, we went looking for flowering coffee. In one corner of the large estate—more than one thousand acres of coffee trees in all—Falla showed me a stand of coffee plants in bloom. Coffee blossoms are white, with slender star shapes, looking much like the serviceberry flowers of the United States. They grow linearly, along the stems. In full flower, they are magnificent, the white flowers contrasting against the deep green, glossy leaves. Of course, these are arabica trees.

It is not just coffee snobs who brag about the origins of their coffee. These days, even diner coffee in the United States is often pure arabica. Dunkin' Donuts, not typically considered an upscale coffeehouse, uses arabica beans exclusively. It sells thirty cups every second, for a total of 1.5 billion cups a year. And McDonald's McCafé coffee is "freshly brewed from a gourmet blend of arabica beans."

These fine coffees inspire lofty praise. For mass-market coffees, we use terms like *bold, smooth, rich*, or *mountain-grown*. For coffee experts, there are more specific terms like *citrus top notes* and *a chocolate finish*.

Coffee experts, like oenophiles, get wacky about "terroir," the idea that certain pieces of ground infuse their products with unique characteristics. Consider this description of a Colombian coffee sold by upmarket Stumptown Coffee Roasters: "Rainier cherry, cranberry, and red apples all provide a counterweight to clover honey and semi-sweet chocolate in this crisp Colombian profile."

Clearly, such coffees are marketed to consumers on the fringe, in terms of the attention they give to flavor and the price they are willing to pay. (Not to mention their tolerance for verbal excess—can anybody really discern Rainier cherry among the cranberry and red apple flavors, or was it perhaps more Bing-like?)

It is true that arabica plants are extremely sensitive, and small changes in temperature and precipitation can have big impacts on coffee quality and quantity, and on flavor. Falla said his farm has a special microclimate. The temperatures rise, more or less, to seventy-nine degrees during the day and fall to fifty degrees at night. This precise range gives his coffee the ideal blend of acidity and flavor. Others agree. Peet's Coffee & Tea claims Falla's is the best farm in the Antigua Valley and gives his coffee this restrained description: "Balanced and refined, yet tantalizingly complex. Hints of bittersweet chocolate."

After our tour, I signed Falla's guest book, then started back to the city. The Volcán de Fuego was sending smoky plumes up into a cloudless sky. And I was thinking about Michael Norton and Kona coffee.

⚡

Coffee flavor gets more complicated when it intersects with the story of a particular coffee. To understand just how important the story is to coffee sales, consider Kona coffee. Grown for generations on the island of Hawaii, the volcanic soils, the balmy temperature, and the tropical rains have helped the coffee develop an excellent reputation as one of the world's finest. The former executive director of the International Coffee Organization, Néstor Osorio, once told me, "Hawaii produces one of the finest coffees in the world." Few coffee lovers would disagree. Its reputation and limited quantity have also made it one of the world's most expensive.

In the mid-1990s, coffee trader Michael Norton saw an opportunity in Kona coffee. Norton was a fixture on the Bay Area coffee scene, sometimes selling bags of green coffee from the back of an old pickup truck. He knew coffee so well, he figured out something that made him millions of dollars.

What Norton understood was that if you looked beyond the Kona label and took away the suggestion of the surf, the Pacific breezes, and Mauna Loa looming nearby, what you had left was a fairly pedestrian brew. A decent coffee, just nothing that would knock your socks off. A coffee, say, like those fair-to-middling Panamanian coffees that wholesaled for less than two dollars per pound.

Norton developed a scheme to import those Central American coffees to Hawaii. In a warehouse there, he hired a shift of workers to empty and sort the coffee. This alone was not unusual. Most Kona coffee is blended, the resulting product containing as little as 10 percent actual Kona coffee. As long as it's marketed as a blend, this is perfectly legit.

But Norton went one step further. He used a separate shift of warehouse workers to re-bag the Panamanian coffee into bags from his Kona Kai Farms. Labeled as Kona coffee from Hawaii, they fetched nearly ten dollars a pound.

Norton laughed all the way to the bank, making $15 million in just a few years. It was a good gig while it lasted. But when a disgruntled employee tipped off the feds, they opened an investigation, complete with wiretaps, video surveillance, and testimony from a guy who used to run hundred-pound bales of weed in a van for Norton, who was ultimately convicted for the scam and sentenced to thirty months in federal prison.

The surprising aspect of the story is that Norton was able to deceive the most educated palates in the business with his faux-Kona coffee, including buyers for Peet's, Starbucks, and Nestlé. But Rhinehart told me that the Norton story is about more than coffee buyers being duped; it is about how we experience and appreciate coffee.

He said coffee is an experiential beverage. "Very, very seldom, if you are not in the business of coffee, do you sit down and analytically taste your coffee," he said. "You drink your coffee." But your perception of that coffee is highly influenced by the context, the place, and the circumstances in which you drink the coffee.

Rhinehart said Kona is a good example. "You wake up in Hawaii, and you look out your window, and it's a beautiful, gorgeous day. It's seventy-two degrees, and the sun is shining. There's a beautiful blue ocean and a nice beach and a person you love lying next to you in bed, and you have a cup of coffee. And that's an exceptional cup of coffee! Regardless of what its absolute quality might be, it's a great cup of coffee."

Rhinehart is right, and it explains why the coffee from Castilla's farm in Colombia was so memorable, even if not a good cup of coffee by modern American standards. But it begs the question, what makes good coffee?

If it's the flavor that makes us wild about coffee, why did our grandparents drink twice as much coffee as we do today? In those days the coffee was often roasted and ground long before it was consumed. And then it was run though a percolator, overextracting the bitter flavors. To most coffee lovers today, our grandparents' coffee was pure percolated plonk. It tasted worse, and they drank twice as much of it.

Yes, there are people with educated palates and extensive cupping experience who really understand flavor. And on the next tier down, there is probably some small percentage of people who appreciate coffee the way a gourmand appreciates food. For the rest of us, it's likely that we are interested not so much in a flavor experience as in a cup of coffee that is, more than anything, unobjectionable. Put another way, we would all prefer a good cup to a mediocre cup. But if the latter is all that is available, we'll damn sure drink it.

If we phrase the question a bit differently—asking not what makes a good cup of coffee, but what makes a cup of coffee good—the answer is easy: caffeine.

But most of us know little about caffeine. Even the most basic coffee distinction—between the robusta beans that become cheap diner coffee and the arabica beans that supply chic coffeehouses—is poorly understood. It's the lowly robusta that packs twice as much caffeine. (Some New York entrepreneurs are turning the notion of premium coffee upside down, selling Death Wish Coffee at a premium because its robusta beans are more caffeinated than arabica beans.) Among the gourmet brews, people commonly perceive that a dark roast, with its strong flavor, has more caffeine than a mild-tasting, light roast. But that, too, is wrong. Because some of the caffeine has been burned off in the longer roasting—actually sublimated as the coffee heats up—darker coffees have less caffeine than light roasts, bean for bean.

Picture a matrix with light roast/dark roast on one axis and gourmet coffee/diner coffee on the other; the least caffeinated of the four is the dark gourmet coffee. Most of us would guess the exact opposite. (Anyone looking for a good caffeine kick might choose a light-roasted Folgers blend.)

So it seems weird—and don't get me wrong; this is not so much sinister as strange—that we lavish so much attention on the other aspects of the coffee experience: the Juan Valdez country-of-origin stories, Howard Schultz's "third place" cafés, and complex flavors. Because, really, they are window dressing. The object of our affection—the drug that makes us energetic, sociable, and happy—is obscured by the stories we tell about coffee.

What we don't talk about when we talk about coffee is the caffeine. And there is plenty to talk about. Bruce Goldberger, the forensic pathologist we met in chapter 2, got his most striking findings when he studied coffee. He and his colleagues bought a variety of coffee drinks and analyzed their caffeine contents, publishing the results in 2003. The caffeine concentrations varied wildly.

Goldberger found that the average caffeine concentration in specialty coffees was twelve milligrams per ounce. This equates to sixty milligrams per five-ounce cup of coffee, which is 40 percent lower than the standard established by a pair of Coca-Cola researchers in an oft-cited paper published in 1996 (they suggested that eighty-five milligrams per five-ounce cup of roasted-and-ground coffee should be the standard). But Goldberger pointed out that while the caffeine content is lower, serving sizes are generally larger. A five-ounce coffee cup is rare, indeed, these days, and a "small" coffee is generally at least ten ounces.

Goldberger found caffeine differences between coffee brands. In his sample, a sixteen-ounce cup of coffee from Dunkin' Donuts had just 143 milligrams of caffeine—less than two Red Bulls, or two SCADs—while a typical cup from Starbucks had twice as much caffeine. Espresso shots appeared to be more consistent in his study, at about seventy-five milligrams of caffeine per single (1.3-ounce) shot.

Goldberger's strangest result came from Starbucks. He bought a sixteen-ounce cup of coffee from one Gainesville Starbucks on six consecutive days. Each time, he ordered the Breakfast Blend, a mixture of Latin American coffees (from farms like Estuardo Falla's San Sebastián). The cup with the least caffeine had 260 milligrams. One cup had twice that amount. Yet another clocked in at a whopping 564 milligrams.

The caffeine varies for several reasons. Brewing strength—the amount of coffee used to prepare a cup—is one variable. The strongest coffee is made using more ground coffee per serving, as opposed to a weak cup of coffee that is as translucent as tea. (This is distinct from the roasting time: both light- and dark-roasted coffees can be brewed on a continuum from weak to strong, depending on the ratio of coffee grounds to water.)

Caffeine also varies because no two plants are exactly alike. Differences in growing conditions and plant variety can lead to dramatically different levels of caffeine.

Following in Goldberger's footsteps, Scottish researcher Thomas Crozier found more evidence of coffee's dramatically varying caffeine levels. For a study published in 2012, Crozier and his colleagues bought twenty espressos in Glasgow cafés. They found that the espressos, all between 0.8 and 2.4 ounces, ranged from 51 to more than 300 milligrams. The caffeine concentration varied from 56 milligrams to 196 milligrams per ounce. This time, Starbucks fell to the bottom of the list; its espresso had just 51 milligrams per 0.9-ounce shot.

Crozier's eyebrow-raising finding was this: A single 1.7-ounce shot of espresso from the Pâtisserie Françoise packed a serious 322 milligrams of caffeine (four SCADs). And it was not much of an outlier: Three other cafés had espressos with more than 200 milligrams of caffeine. Crozier wrote, "The levels of caffeine per serving varied more than 6-fold from 51 to 322 mg. At the low level, a pregnant woman and others with a need to restrict caffeine consumption, might safely drink 4 cups per day without significantly exceeding the recommended caffeine intake. In marked contrast, at the higher end of the scale, drinking even one cup of espresso will be well in excess of the advised limit of 200 mg day."

Starbucks seems unperturbed by the dramatically varying caffeine levels. On its Web site, it simply notes that its brewed coffees have twenty milligrams of caffeine per ounce, making no reference to this well-documented variability.

The studies by Crozier and Goldberger help to answer a question that many coffee drinkers have asked: Why is it that on some days one cup of coffee puts you in absolute equipoise—brilliant but steady, relaxed but energetic—while other days it is not even enough to prop open your eyelids? And on still other occasions, that very same cup—

the same size, the same blend, from the same café—will send you to the moon, jittery and anxious, your heart skittering or pounding? It is because the caffeine levels in coffee vary dramatically, depending on the natural growing conditions, the variety of coffee plant, and brewing strength. To contrast it with a common delivery system of another well-loved drug, alcohol, it would be as if one bottle of wine delivered the expected 13 percent alcohol and another delivered five times as much, a dose stronger than gin, rum, or whiskey.

Much of the Guatemala conference focused on the threats facing coffee due to a changing climate and shifting demand. But Judy Ganes-Chase, a consultant from New York, mentioned another threat. She said that energy drinks are not just siphoning off caffeine drinkers; they're evolving into strange coffee-flavored hybrids. Canned products like Rockstar Roasted and Java Monster blend the energy drink concept that Americans imported from Indonesia with the canned coffee the Japanese have popularized. They are basically coffee drinks juiced with added caffeine.

Ganes-Chase noted that such drinks blur the regulatory boundaries as health advocates call for better caffeine labeling on energy drinks, while coffee already walks a fine line between a drink and a drug. "I think it's a very dangerous line because you don't want to worry about labeling issues," she said.

Just outside the convention center was a billboard advertising an energy drink, Pepsi Kick, with caffeine and ginseng. It showed roosters crowing into the ears of a sleepy man. "¡Despierta!" the billboard shouted, "Wake up!" It was a message equally suited to the coffee traditionalists at the conference, because the industry is evolving so rapidly that the traditional coffeepot may soon look as archaic as a horse and buggy. Much of the evolution has been driven by one New England company that has changed Americans' coffee habits, a single serving at a time.

CHAPTER 4

Building a Better Cup of Coffee

ob Stiller is the sort of person you might see in a Vermont co-op and think he's been out in the woods too long. He fits the bill to a degree, inclined as he is toward wooly sweaters, meditation, yoga, and the New Age philosophy of Deepak Chopra. But his laid-back demeanor belies the mind of a sharp capitalist. By 2011, he had used his business savvy to accrue a billion-dollar fortune. He split his time between a Palm Beach mansion, a 150-foot yacht, and the $17 million Columbus Circle condo he bought from Tom Brady and Giselle Bündchen. He was the single largest shareholder of Krispy Kreme. But Stiller is best known for something else entirely: He founded one of the most innovative and profitable coffee companies in the world.

A cup of coffee quite literally changed Stiller's life. That was in 1980, when he was at loose ends, a thirty-seven-year-old entrepreneur with $3 million burning a hole in his pocket after selling his first company. He was living in a condo at Sugarbush, a Vermont ski area, when he stumbled onto an exceptionally tasty brew in nearby Waitsfield. Stiller was so inspired by that experience that he bought the tiny coffee company and began growing it, in the shaggy, green-tinged style of Ben & Jerry's. That was the creation of Green Mountain Coffee Roasters.

Stiller became obsessed with coffee, roasting small batches at home using cookie sheets and popcorn poppers. It goes without saying that he used arabica beans exclusively. In 1980, many Americans were like Stiller—they had never tasted a fresh, well-made cup of arabica, only overcooked percolator coffee or instant coffee. So he had a jump-start on the nascent boom in gourmet coffee.

The timing was right for gourmet coffee roasters to introduce some competition into the coffee industry. Commercial coffee was then being roasted very lightly, partly because the robusta in the blends tastes especially bad at darker roasts. Against the backdrop of those light-roast commercial coffees, the darker-roast coffees popularized by Peet's Coffee and Starbucks were quickly able to distinguish themselves. Ric Rhinehart said the formula was simple: "Roast the coffee darker, bring out these chocolate tones and some of the caramelized sweetness notes that people like, and brew it strong, and let people drink it."

Demand for gourmet coffee was just starting to grow like wildfire. Starbucks was putting America at the epicenter of the gourmet coffee revolution by developing a chain of cafés selling coffee that was consistently strong and dark . . . and expensive. Stiller's small, regional company was swept along as American coffee tastes changed, and Green Mountain's coffee bean sales grew steadily.

By 1997, though, Stiller had a problem. Green Mountain sales had slowed after years of steady growth. Stiller saw that despite the conspicuous embrace of gourmet roasts that had pulled coffee out of its decades-long decline, Americans' appetites for the caffeinated beverage were growing very slowly.

Starbucks was leading the modern coffee revolution by doing what American companies do best—applying McDonald's-style convenience, standardization, and supersizing to lattes and cappuccinos. But the Starbucks model wasn't working for Green Mountain. Starbucks had fourteen hundred cafés in 1997, while Green Mountain's chain of less than a dozen cafés was losing money so quickly that they threatened to sink the entire company. Green Mountain could either remain a healthy niche coffee company, popular in New England and little-known elsewhere, or it could innovate and claw some of that market share away from its competitors in the supersaturated coffee market.

Stiller needed to find his own distinctly American way to serve coffee. His business savvy and market intuition helped him understand one simple concept that eventually would make him one of the richest men in the country: Most Americans prefer their coffee in frequent, fresh, strong doses, often on the run. Stiller decided that if people would not come to his cafés, he would take his coffee to them, wherever they were. He set out to infiltrate convenience store chains, which then mostly served stale, burnt, or weak coffee from sad-looking glass pots. Hundreds of New England ExxonMobil stores soon were dispensing Green Mountain coffee from vacuum pump pots, bringing premium coffee to the masses. Distinctive signs in front of the convenience stores advertised Green Mountain coffee, a jarring but welcome contrast for those who associated gourmet coffee only with funky cafés.

To understand Green Mountain's next innovation, it is helpful to know that Stiller had already demonstrated some mastery of single-serving packages. In the early 1970s, he and a partner had been frustrated by a problem endemic to the era: Cigarette papers were too narrow for rolling joints. Like other stoners, they usually solved the problem by gluing two papers together. But they also saw it as a business opportunity and launched a brand that anyone who attended college and actually did inhale will recognize: the rolling paper company called E-Z Wider. Their innovation was to supersize cigarette rolling papers to make it easier to roll fat joints. In 1980, they sold ninety-one million packs—enough to roll two billion joints—and then sold the company. They parted ways, each pocketing $3.1 million. That's how Stiller made the money that staked him to his Green Mountain gambit.

Extending his knack for micro-packaging and his intuition for gaps in the market, Stiller took the idea of dispensing convenience one step further, seeing sooner and better than anyone else at the top of the American coffee industry that the trend for coffee drinkers was toward single-serve doses. In offices throughout the world, that nasty pot of burnt coffee in the break room was going the way of the dinosaur. And his great innovation was to find, buy, and promote the Keurig system, with its single-serving coffee pods.

⚡

Stiller's crunchy little coffee roasting company now occupies a sprawling campus in Waterbury, a town nestled in a mountain valley between Burlington and Montpelier. The roasting plant has the eighteen-wheelers and loading docks of any industrial facility. But the trucks run on biodiesel and the warehouse roof is covered with solar panels. Trees line the parking lots, and green hills roll up to the horizon in all directions. Often enveloped in the aroma of roasting coffee, it has a mellow vibe that feels more like a college campus than a food-processing plant.

In the visitor's center, a beautifully renovated train depot, you can sip a cup of fresh-brewed coffee while perusing elaborate displays about Green Mountain's environmental commitment and its links to coffee farmers. You can see many variants of the classic photo of work-hardened hands cupping coffee beans. If you did not know better, it might seem more like the headquarters of a nonprofit designed to improve conditions for workers in developing countries and protect the environment.

Back in the business end of the operation, in a huge warehouse with an earthy smell, green coffee beans are stacked high overhead in thousands of sixty-kilo burlap sacks. These are raw coffee beans, loaded into bags overseas and then manually stacked onto pallets by strong men working in tandem, with cargo hooks in each hand, piercing, swinging, and heaving the heavy bags. That is the primitive side of Green Mountain's operation.

Stepping from the warehouse into an adjacent building where the beans are roasted, ground, and packed is like stepping from *Oliver Twist* into *The Matrix*. The beating heart of the Green Mountain plant is a building filled with gleaming, sanitized assembly lines that pump out billions of K-Cups annually.

K-Cups look like oversize creamer tubs. On special machines here, the plastic cups are lined with paper filters, filled with coffee, topped off with nitrogen to prevent oxidation, and sealed with foil.

It is worth pausing here to consider the nitrogen. By producing K-Cups, Green Mountain is committing heresy in gourmet coffee circles. Coffee aficionados agree on two key steps in brewing excellent coffee: using coffee that is freshly roasted and grinding it shortly before you prepare it. Once you grind the coffee, the volatile oils start to depart (that wonderful smell of freshly ground coffee is the flavor taking wing and wafting away). Oxygen then infiltrates the coffee, oxidizing it, bringing off-flavors, and often bitterness, to the product.

This is not a bit of late-breaking news from the coffee frontiers, just standard coffee knowledge passed down through the generations. Consider this passage, from an 1896 military report discussing the difficulties of getting good coffee to soldiers in the field:

> It has been stated by coffee experts that roasted coffee, especially when ground, will not keep in any method of preparation known. Even hermetically sealing is not a perfect means of preserving it and firms dealing in this article have stated that in the course of a few months the coffee deteriorates or "sours," the ground coffee sooner than the unground. They state that the total exclusion of air being impossible without ruining the coffee in the processing, the sealing of the package excluding more air from entering only delays the deterioration a few months.

By displacing the oxygen in its K-Cups with nitrogen, Green Mountain Coffee Roasters avoids the problem of oxidation. A steady stream of K-Cups blasts through the line in a mesmerizing synchronized flow, each packing precisely eleven grams of ground coffee. Convenient single servings of America's favorite caffeinated beverage. High-tech marvels. One-hit wonders.

In a Keurig machine, pins puncture the foil top and plastic bottom of the K-Cup, and hot water flows through, brewing a drink directly into a mug waiting below. It is a quick and easy single serving of coffee. Green Mountain sold three billion of the pods in 2010 alone.

Keurig, a Massachusetts company, is a wholly owned subsidiary of Green Mountain. Following the same model as Hewlett-Packard, which sells cheap printers but makes huge profits on the print cartridges, or Gillette, which uses the same model to sell inexpensive razors with pricey replacement blades, Green Mountain is able to keep Keurig machine costs low. The machines, made in China, start at less than $100, often bundled with a starter pack of a dozen K-Cups. Still, machine sales netted the company more than $200 million in 2010. But the K-Cup is the product that took Green Mountain from an eco-friendly regional company to a Wall Street darling. Its stock price quadrupled between 2007 and 2010. If you'd had the prescience to invest $1,000 in the company when it went public in 1993, you would have made $20 million by the fall of 2011. (Didn't have $1,000 to invest in 1993? On an investment of just $100, you would have made $2 million. Try not to cry.) Between 2006 and 2011, the stock—GMCR on NASDAQ—did better than Apple, Google, and even Starbucks.

In offices, where the Keurig machines first took root soon after their introduction in 2003, coworkers no longer had to complain that someone had made coffee that was too weak or too strong, too light or too dark, or that the coffee had been simmering for hours into a bitter, burnt sludge. People could pop their own pods on demand. The K-Cup was taking the coffee market by storm.

The little Vermont company was competing with global food giants for the coffee pod market, and winning. Nestlé was in the game with its Dolce Gusto coffee system and upscale Nespresso espresso machines. Mars had Flavia, and Kraft had Tassimo. Sara Lee had Senseo. All used proprietary coffee pods.

By 2010, Green Mountain claimed double-digit growth each quarter for seven and a half years, most driven by K-Cups, which comprised 86 percent of its sales. By 2011, Green Mountain was filling its thimbles for Dunkin' Donuts. Newman's Own Organics K-Cups quickly became the top-selling item for that company, founded by Paul Newman's daughter to promote organic foods. (Ironically, Nell Newman, an ardent environmentalist, saw her company's sales led by a product that is non-recyclable and non-compostable).

Another coffee giant took a run at the single-serve market from a different direction. Starbucks introduced its Via instant coffee in single-serving tubes in February 2009; by year's end, sales had reached $50 million. But Starbucks, too, saw the allure of the K-Cup. Green Mountain stock jumped 42 percent in one day in March 2011, when it announced an agreement to package Starbucks coffee in K-Cups. That jump launched Stiller onto the 2011 Forbes list of richest Americans, with an estimated worth of $1.3 billion. By a strange coincidence, he was tied for 331st place on the list with Starbucks CEO Howard Schultz.

A single K-Cup costs about ninety cents. That's a reasonable price for a cup of coffee, but it works out to thirty dollars per pound. Put another way, Green Mountain's coffees are selling for more per pound than the farm-specific beans sold to coffee snobs by Intelligentsia, Stumptown, and the like. What's even more remarkable is that Green Mountain is getting these highbrow prices in mass-market retailers— supermarket chains and Sam's Clubs.

This is Stiller's great innovation, using the alchemy of the marketplace to nearly triple the per-pound price of Green Mountain coffee while creating skyrocketing demand. The whole model is based on making it quick and easy to get a tasty caffeine jolt.

Green Mountain has stopped listing the number of K-Cups it sells (perhaps due to some ugly shareholder lawsuits), but it's likely that they sold about six billion in 2011. To put this in perspective, the 2011 production of K-Cups, lined up end-to-end, would encircle the equator six times—a foot-wide belt of plastic, foil, and coffee around the planet.

⚡

Stiller's days among the richest Americans ended two ways, to paraphrase Hemingway: gradually and then all of a sudden. Green Mountain shares hit their apex of $111.62 on September 19, 2011. Investors marveled at the stock's high returns, and the business press made punny headlines, playing on "coffee high" and the like. But the stock seemed overvalued to some. In October, the influential hedge fund manager David Einhorn spent an hour critiquing the company at an investors' conference, alleging questionable accounting practices. The day after his presentation, shares started falling. After a poor earnings report in November, they fell further, to below fifty dollars. Soon the Louisiana Municipal Police Employees' Retirement System, which had invested in the company, sued Green Mountain over their losses.

The company's next challenge came not from jilted investors, but from an aggressive competitor. On March 8, 2012, Green Mountain shares fell ten dollars from their current price of $62.59, when Starbucks announced it was developing its own pod system. (Remember Green Mountain's stock jump after its Starbucks announcement, just a year earlier.) That alone was bad news for investors. But then it got worse: Investors learned that Stiller had dumped $66 million in stock, his biggest sale ever, a few days before the announcement.

As Stiller's portfolio plummeted in value and his credibility as a CEO tanked, worse news, yet, was coming. On May 3, after a poor earnings report, Green Mountain shares lost half their value in a single day, falling to $25.87 a share. And this is where it gets strange. It turned out that Stiller had borrowed heavily against his shares, and his nervous creditors at Deutsche Bank made a margin call when the stock plunged. Stiller sold five million shares of Green Mountain stock on Monday, May 7, cashing out for $123 million. He made the trade during a standard, company-imposed blackout period bracketing the quarterly earnings reports, when insiders were not supposed to trade. The board of directors hastily arranged a phone meeting. By Tuesday, they had voted him out as chairman.

It was a surprisingly desperate tear for the mellow entrepreneur. Not only did Stiller lose three-quarters of his worth in just nine months; he lost leadership of the company he'd founded and led for three decades.

But Green Mountain has regained its stability, and it still owes its success to Stiller's innovations. In his E-Z Wider days, Stiller demonstrated a knack for selling convenient single-serving packaging for popular drugs. With Green Mountain, he went one better. He figured out how to sell the drug itself—one that most Americans take daily and hope never to have to go without. And he did this in a way that is not just legal, but culturally accepted, convenient, and wildly profitable. It is a hell of a business model, and it sure beats selling rolling papers.

Stiller has done well by marijuana and coffee. "I know people might think they're drugs, but I really look on them as products," he said in an interview with *Vermont Business Magazine*. "And I try to provide the best quality coffee, as I tried to produce the best quality paper. With the papers, it was a limited market. I love that the coffee market is so huge."

Call it a product or call it a drug, this is one of the victories of modern technology and a global economy. Anyone, anywhere in the United States, can pop a thimble into a machine, pull the lever, and make a fine, single cup of Colombian coffee that's packing a solid two SCADs. It matters not that it was harvested thousands of miles away on a farm like Castilla's. Even after being shipped across the Caribbean and up the Mississippi, warehoused, trucked to Vermont, ground, packed, and sent off to another warehouse, to stores like Sam's Club, and finally to your coffee cup, it has lost little of its flavor and little of its caffeine (though more than Green Mountain would like, I later discovered).

By packaging his caffeine into convenient single servings, Stiller made it easier than ever to get a tasty cup of coffee with a solid dose of caffeine. Pop in the cup and pull down the lever. A monkey could do it. And probably would.

CHAPTER 5

Pulling the Lever

Long before K-Cups came onto the scene, a dogged scientist in Baltimore was starting to understand why such a device might become so popular. Roland Griffiths is a prolific drug researcher. A few pieces of framed art hang on the walls of his spare office at Johns Hopkins Bayview Medical Center—a vintage Coca-Cola ad, a copy of the cartoon *Too Much Coffee Man*, and a Bruce Nauman poster titled "Caffeine Dreams." A shelf above his desk holds a long row of books on coffee and caffeine. But a row of filing cabinets that occupies one wall best illustrates the depth and breadth of Griffiths's research.

The block of cabinets is three drawers tall and five wide. Ten of the fifteen drawers are labeled CAFFEINE. The other five are labeled PSILO-CYBIN (his work on "magic mushrooms" as a tool to fight depression has been covered in the *New York Times*).

"I'm a psychopharmcologist, so I'm interested in mood-altering effects of drugs," Griffiths told me. "For the past forty years I've studied, in animals and humans, various psychoactive drugs. Caffeine to me is one of the most fascinating, maybe the most fascinating compound. Because it clearly is psychoactive, and yet it is completely culturally accepted worldwide, or almost worldwide."

Griffiths is a tall, slender man with short white hair. He has an easy smile that gives his eyes a twinkle behind his spectacles. He listens closely to questions, giving the impression he is really paying attention, and when he replies, he speaks thoughtfully and precisely. While we talked, he sipped caffeine-free Diet Coke from a mug bearing the structural diagram of the caffeine molecule.

He told me that most drug research is aimed at problematic drugs of abuse. So he became interested in studying the world's most widely consumed psychoactive drug. Even though it's not considered to be a drug of abuse in virtually any culture, it has all the features of a drug of abuse. "That is, it alters mood, it produces physical dependence, it produces withdrawal upon abstinence, and some proportion of the population becomes dependent on it," said Griffiths.

Caffeine gave Griffiths a model system for understanding the interactions between behavior and abusable drugs, and one he could study without the ethical restraints that face researchers studying drugs like cocaine and heroin.

He rummaged through the file drawers for a few minutes, then brought over a paper titled "Human Coffee Drinking: Manipulation of Concentration and Caffeine Dose." "This is how I got into the caffeine work," said Griffiths. "This was our first study where we just started to look at cups of coffee consumed across the day." In other words, this is the study that kicked off more than a quarter century of caffeine research.

For that early research, Griffiths and his colleagues studied nine subjects, all male, all heavy coffee drinkers. In double-blind conditions (meaning neither the subjects nor the researchers administering the dose knew what the dose contained), the coffee drinkers were allowed to drink coffee "ad libitum" (at will), while Griffiths manipulated the coffee strength and caffeine levels.

For starters, it seemed that nearly everyone had a similar pattern, one that most coffee drinkers will recognize. In the morning, subjects had several cups of coffee at short intervals. As the day progressed, the cups of coffee became fewer and farther between. When they were given stronger coffee (a more concentrated brew), the subjects decreased their coffee consumption, although they continued to space it out over the day. And when the researchers increased the caffeine levels but did not increase the coffee strength, they saw a similar effect.

In all, wrote Griffiths, "The present set of studies has revealed coffee drinking to be a stable and orderly form of drug self-administration behavior that is readily amenable to experimental analysis using intensive in-subject experimental design."

OK, there's a bit of research jargon there, but that sentence includes a very concise description of something that most American adults do every day, by referring to coffee drinking as "a stable and orderly form of drug self-administration."

Griffiths told me the patterns of self-administration he saw in human coffee drinkers in that early study looked quite familiar: they looked like the patterns he'd seen in his lab studies on animals.

Self-administration is a pretty basic concept. Rig up a lab rat with an IV tube connected to a pump with, say, a pleasure-inducing opiate. Then place a lever in the cage that the rat can press to get a dose of the drug. When the rat presses the lever, it is self-administering drugs. Scientists count the number of times the animal presses the lever and the intervals between doses. "Likewise, coffee drinking can be viewed as a form of drug self-administration," Griffiths said, "and you can measure sips or cups of coffee per day." As that early study showed, the subjects were reliably dosing themselves with their preferred amount of caffeine and adjusting the timing and amount of coffee consumption to attain that optimal dose.

We are not talking about opiates here, but by looking at coffee drinking with Griffiths's research in mind, you'll see more than people stumbling to the coffeepot first thing in the morning or strolling to the break room at ten a.m. or the café at lunchtime. You'll see hundreds of millions of lab rats, systematically and repeatedly pushing the buttons on Coke machines or pulling the levers on Keurig machines, self-administering doses of caffeine.

From that early research, Griffiths went on to conduct an elegant series of studies, methodically examining human interactions with the drug caffeine. Over the years, he studied self-administration, reinforcement, discrimination, tolerance, and dependence and withdrawal. It's worth taking some time to understand the terminology here, since for people who use caffeine regularly, these terms describe the behaviors that structure our days.

Reinforcement is a trigger that increases the likelihood you will engage in that behavior again. If you drink a Pepsi, say, and it makes you feel good, you will probably do it again.

To test reinforcement, you give subjects the choice among several items—it could be a cola or coffee or a capsule—over a period of days or weeks. One of the choices is a placebo; the other is caffeinated. The subjects don't know which is which. If over time they show a distinct preference for, say, the yellow capsule over the orange capsule, the caffeinated over the uncaffeinated product, this shows that caffeine functions as a reinforcer.

Griffiths said the term is especially useful in cases in which people are not aware that their behavior is being driven by a drug. He said many people used to be unaware that caffeine underlies their consumption habits, and some still are. "They would make the attribution based on the taste of coffee in the morning, or they've always had a cup of coffee with their newspaper, and they just like doing that, and they could take or leave the caffeine," he said.

Reinforcement is not the same as euphoria. A large dose of caffeine will give you a good kick and often a sense of euphoria. But reinforcement is often much more subtle, occurring below the level of consciousness.

Discrimination is the ability to subjectively detect the presence of a compound. To test this, researchers might give someone a capsule that has either caffeine or a placebo and check to see if that person is able to detect the presence or absence of caffeine, and at what level.

Tolerance we all understand. It is the body's ability to become less responsive to a certain dose of a drug through exposure. When it comes to caffeine, most of us tend to develop partial tolerance. So if you use caffeine regularly, you get much less of a kick from your daily cup of coffee than from the first cup you ever tasted. The key mechanism at work here is that habitual caffeine users develop more adenosine receptors, in an effort to skirt caffeine's adenosine-blocking effects. Scientists call this "up-regulation." (With abstinence, it likely takes about a week for adenosine receptors to reset to a baseline level, though it might take longer.)

Now, finally, to addiction and withdrawal. This is where Griffiths's research gets personal. When Griffiths started his experiments on caffeine, he was a heavy caffeine user. "I think my consumption was probably, I would guess, five hundred to six hundred milligrams a day, maybe higher," he told me. That's more than seven SCADs. It's seven Red Bulls. Or thirty-six ounces of good coffee.

When he decided to study caffeine withdrawal, he did it the hard way. Griffiths and six colleagues participated in a series of studies on caffeine. "They are unusual papers because the authors are also the subjects," he told me. For his part, that meant going from a daily dose of seven to eight SCADs down to zero and paying close attention to the havoc it wreaked on his body and brain.

I asked Griffiths if he went cold turkey. "No, no!" he said. "I'm enough of a psychopharmacologist to know that's not how I would want to do it. I tapered back."

Griffiths and his colleagues were not the first to quit caffeine in the name of science. William Halse Rivers Rivers, a well-born British doctor and adventuring anthropologist, had also done some research on caffeine in humans. His book *The Influence of Alcohol and Other Drugs on Fatigue*, based on lectures he delivered in 1906, surveyed then-recent caffeine research and documented his own studies.

"I began my work on drugs with an experiment on the effects of caffeine, and discontinued the use of tea and coffee shortly before the experiment began, having previously taken them in diminished quantity," he said in a lecture on caffeine. "The act of giving up those substances was followed by loss of energy, which greatly interfered with the success of the experiment, and a later repetition of the experience left little doubt that the condition was due, at any rate in part, to the discontinuance of the use of coffee and tea."

Rivers stopped taking any caffeine or alcohol for an entire year before subjecting himself to experiments. With dry understatement, he noted that few researchers would likely follow his lead: "So drastic a procedure is not likely to attract workers to this subject."

But eight decades later, Griffiths et al. were, indeed, attracted to this subject. In the first in a series of studies using themselves as guinea pigs, Griffiths and his colleagues slowly reduced their caffeine consumption. Along the way, they conducted discrimination tests to see if they could tell the difference between caffeine and placebo capsules. (All of these tests were conducted double-blind.)

Not surprisingly, they were all able to reliably tell the difference between a placebo and one hundred milligrams or more of caffeine. And it was not as obvious as it sounds. The caffeine was not administered in a single one-hundred-milligram bump, which would have been easy to detect, but in ten 10-milligram capsules spaced out over the day.

The researchers wrote, "Compared to placebo, 100 mg of caffeine increased ratings of alertness, well-being, social disposition, motivation for work, concentration, energy, and self-confidence, and decreased ratings of headache and sleepiness. This dose of caffeine also produced a measure of 'euphoria.'"

A more surprising finding, in a second phase of the discrimination experiment, was that some subjects had a very low threshold for detecting caffeine. All of the seven subjects could easily detect less than a SCAD: Three were able to detect fifty-six milligrams of caffeine (the amount in a twelve-ounce Mountain Dew); three could detect eighteen milligrams of caffeine (half the amount in a can of Coke); and one was able to notice just ten milligrams. (In a later study, Griffiths found that a subject was able to detect a mere 3.2 milligrams of caffeine—a tiny sip of coffee, or a tenth of a can of Coke.)

From this study, the scientists—all now on a steady maintenance dose of one hundred milligrams of caffeine daily—moved on to studying dependence. This time they tried to understand withdrawal in two ways. First, they substituted placebo capsules for caffeine for twelve consecutive days, going from daily doses of one hundred milligrams of caffeine to none. Again, the capsules were administered double-blind, and the subjects were not told when their caffeine was being cut.

In this phase, four of the seven subjects experienced "an orderly withdrawal syndrome." The symptoms included headaches, lethargy, and an inability to concentrate. "The syndrome peaked on days 1 or 2 and progressively decreased toward pre-withdrawal levels over about 1 week," they wrote.

In the second phase, the researchers substituted placebos for caffeine for one-day intervals, separated by more than a week. In this case, "each of the seven subjects demonstrated a statistically significant withdrawal effect."

Again, these scientists were not withdrawing from massive doses of caffeine, just one hundred milligrams daily. This is the amount in about five to eight ounces of coffee, two cans of Diet Coke, or three cans of Coke. Perhaps two or three cups of tea. A SCAD and a third. That is all it takes to get hooked. (It may take even less, Griffiths told me, but there is not yet research that has tested this.)

In their paper, the scientists wrote:

> Although the phenomenon of caffeine withdrawal has been described previously, the present report documents that the incidence of caffeine withdrawal is higher (100% of subjects), the daily dose level at which withdrawal occurs is lower (roughly equivalent to the amount of caffeine

in a single cup of brewed coffee or three cans of caffeinated
soft drink), and the range of symptoms experienced is
broader (including headache, fatigue, and other dysphoric
mood changes, muscle pain/stiffness, flu-like feelings,
nausea/vomiting and craving for caffeine) than heretofore
recognized.

This paper stirred the hornet's nest. Given that most American
adults take caffeine daily, and the average intake is well above one hundred milligrams, the research suggested that most of us would experience some real unpleasantness if we abruptly stopped taking the
drug. How much? Griffiths took that up in a later paper, a 2004 literature review. Here he found that half of all experimental subjects reported headaches upon caffeine withdrawal, and fully 13 percent
reported "clinically significant distress or functional impairment."

So let's think about this more broadly. Let's say the American caffeine supply chain were to be abruptly disrupted, and none of us could
have caffeine tomorrow. Or that, for some reason, we were to celebrate
a National No-Caffeine Day, analogous to the Great American Smoke-
out. Since about 80 percent of Americans take caffeine daily, these results suggest that 125 million people would be walking around with
headaches, and 32 million of us—nearly the entire population of
California—would be experiencing significant distress or functional
impairment.

Taken together, Griffiths's studies paint a picture of a drug that is
not just attractive, but addictive. "When I first used the word 'addiction'
with respect to caffeine, the industry came down on me like crazy," Griffiths said with a chuckle. "But I don't have any problem in saying that
caffeine is a mildly addicting drug. I think that describes it."

But some scientists challenge the label "addictive" for caffeine.
Carlton Erickson, a University of Texas professor of pharmacology
and toxicology, once wrote, "To suggest that caffeine 'addiction' somehow belongs in the same category as cocaine addiction, heroin addic-

tion, alcohol addiction, and nicotine addiction gives the term 'addiction' a bad name. We have enough stigma in this field without labeling all overuse of any chemical or any 'I really like it' activity as an addiction." Erickson said withdrawal and tolerance do not constitute addiction.

Dr. Sally Satel is also skeptical. Her 2006 literature review is titled "Is Caffeine Addictive?" And her answer? No. Satel acknowledged that coffee drinking (not caffeine use) is "weakly reinforcing" and wrote, "The possible reinforcing effects of coffee may not be the caffeine per se, but rather the pleasurable aroma and taste of coffee as well as the social environment that usually accompanies coffee consumption." And she has a phrase for this sort of coffee consumption: "In short, coffee drinking resembles more a dedicated habit than a compulsive addiction."

Satel also critiqued the methodologies behind several caffeine studies. In sum, she found, "The common-sense use of the term addiction is that regular consumption is irresistible and that it creates problems. Caffeine use does not fit this profile."

Satel is a resident scholar at the American Enterprise Institute, a conservative think tank. Her research was funded by the American Beverage Association, which represents the soft-drink industry and has long fought regulations for caffeine. So a skeptical observer would suspect her to be disinclined to find caffeine addictive. Even so, her conclusion was less compelling because it included this proviso: "Though cessation of regular use may result in symptoms such as headache and lethargy, these are easily and reliably reversed by ingestion of caffeine. Avoidance of such symptoms, when they do occur, is easily accomplished by ingesting successively smaller doses of caffeine over about a week-long period." Including these instructions for dealing with withdrawal makes Satel's argument against the addictive qualities of caffeine seem a bit less persuasive, more nuanced.

In their literature review, Griffiths and coauthor Laura Juliano argued that caffeine withdrawal should be added to the caffeine-related disorders listed in the *Diagnostic and Statistical Manual of Psychiatric Disorders*. The manual, better known as the DSM, is a doorstop of a diagnostic tool. First published in 1953, and regularly revised, it is the American Psychiatric Association's effort to classify mental disorders.

The revised DSM published in 2000 included four caffeine-induced disorders. The disorder known as "caffeine intoxication" is what it sounds like: restlessness, nervousness, insomnia, intestinal distress, rambling thoughts or speech, or rapid heartbeats. "Caffeine-induced anxiety disorder" is diagnosed when caffeine causes anxiety, panic attacks, or obsessive or compulsive behavior. "Caffeine-induced sleep disorder" needs little description. And the DSM also listed "caffeine-related disorder not otherwise specified."

Griffiths's efforts paid off. The DSM-5, the major revision released in 2013, finally included a diagnosis of "caffeine withdrawal." This puts caffeine on a par with other drugs whose withdrawal the DSM recognizes as unique diagnoses: cocaine, nicotine, and opiates. The caffeine withdrawal diagnosis must include cessation or reduction in caffeine intake, followed by several symptoms such as headache, fatigue, irritability, depressed mood, nausea, and muscle pain.

Griffiths also urged the American Psychiatric Association to include a diagnosis of "caffeine dependence" under its addiction criteria in the DSM. He acknowledged that this is fraught, because there is a concern that caffeine dependence could be overdiagnosed. And if any psychological disorder is overdiagnosed, you run the risk of trivializing the DSM.

Ever methodical, Griffiths conducted research on caffeine dependence, to see if it really does exist as a condition that can be consistently diagnosed. He and his colleagues advertised to find people who felt they were "psychologically or physically dependent on caffeine" or had "tried unsuccessfully to quit using caffeinated products in the past."

They recruited ninety-four people who met the criteria. The subjects filled out questionnaires about their medical histories and caffeine consumption patterns. No surprises here: The subjects, on average, consumed about 550 milligrams daily (more than seven SCADs). But a quarter of them used less than 289 milligrams daily. They tended to use a variety of caffeinated products: Coffee was the primary source of caffeine for half of the subjects, a third preferred soft drinks, and a handful, just one in twenty, primarily consumed tea.

In their 2012 paper, Griffiths and his colleagues wrote, "The most common reason offered by participants for wanting to quit or reduce caffeine consumption were general or specific health concerns. . . . Interestingly, some participants reported that they viewed caffeine modification as a means to lose weight because their caffeinated beverages of choice were sugary soft drinks."

When the researchers applied DSM substance-abuse criteria to the caffeine users, 93 percent met the diagnosis. But Griffiths told me he recommended counting something as a caffeine-use disorder only if a person meets three supplemental criteria: persistent desire or unsuccessful efforts to cut down or control; continued use despite knowledge of having a persistent or recurring physical or psychological problem likely caused or exacerbated by caffeine use; and experiencing withdrawal, or continuing to use to avoid withdrawal.

But it's not as simple as just having these problems, said Griffiths. The diagnosis also requires that these are patterns of caffeine use "leading to clinically significant impairment or distress."

This all sounds a bit technical, but Griffiths said the basic criteria are pretty simple: "The core ones are this persistent desire or inability to quit, and using despite having a medical or psychological problem. And for me, if you have both of those, I mean, that's what addiction is: You want to quit, you have a reason to quit, and you can't, and you've tried." He acknowledges that caffeine dependence is vastly different from better known addictions. "One of the features of caffeine as you run the dose up is initially there are positive effects, but you run headlong into adverse effects," he said. "As you raise the dose of caffeine, you run into anxiety, jitteriness, and stomach upset. Much in the same way as you do with nicotine if you run the dose up." This gives caffeine and nicotine a sort of self-limiting feature and is one of the key distinctions between these drugs and the more classic drugs of abuse like opiates and amphetamines. Going back to the early experiments on self-administration, most caffeine users tend to find a dose and consumption pattern that suits them and stick with it.

Griffiths was disappointed that caffeine use disorder was not included in the DSM-5, but it may be on the way for the next revision. It's listed in the new manual as an issue deserving further research, which is often an interim step to a future diagnosis—caffeine withdrawal lived in those back pages in the previous edition of the DSM.

Most people would draw a hard line between caffeine addiction and, say, opiate addiction. Caffeine addicts may do some crazy things to grab a much-needed cup of joe, but they don't tend to knock over drugstores and banks to feed their jones. Still, there are some peculiar links between caffeine and other drugs of abuse.

Caffeine is one of the most popular cutting agents for heroin and has been for years. A 1972 House Committee on Foreign Affairs report stated, "Analysis of the so-called Red Rock heroin available in Vietnam shows it to contain 3 to 4% heroin, 3 to 4% strychnine, and 32% caffeine as active ingredients. A concentration this low would be known as 'junk.'"

Besides the fact that it is a cheap, white powder, there may be other reasons for cutting heroin with caffeine. According to the Counter Narcotics Police of Afghanistan, "Users who smoke or inhale heroin draw some practical benefits if it is mixed with a certain amount of caffeine, as this causes the heroin to vaporize at a lower temperature."

Caffeine is such a popular cutting agent that a pair of British men were convicted for drug trafficking even though they had only legal drugs—acetaminophen and caffeine. By proving that the men brought 150 kilos of the drugs into England (at Dover Docks, in a white VW van) for the purpose of cutting heroin, prosecutors were able to put them in jail for eight years.

The U.S. Drug Enforcement Administration's *Microgram Bulletin*, a roundup of drug busts, regularly features seizures of various drugs adulterated with caffeine. Some Medusa ecstasy tablets seized in California in 2003 were reported to contain 95 percent caffeine and just 4 percent of the MDMA that gives ecstasy its psychoactive properties. The DEA also regularly nabs cocaine that has been cut with caffeine and fake OxyContin pills that have been blended with caffeine.

A kitchen chemist looking for a stronger caffeine buzz has even posted an online tutorial for making "black magic," smokable caffeine. It's a freebase analogue made on a stovetop, by cooking condensed coffee with ammonia. Stoners who enjoy smoking weed while drinking a strong cup of coffee call the combination a "hippie speedball." It's not quite the cocaine-heroin combination of the original speedball, but it's probably not a smart choice: Research in rats showed that the combination of THC (the primary active ingredient in marijuana) and caffeine impaired memory more than marijuana does alone. The combo might make you dazed and confused, but it's not likely to kill you, either, as an actual speedball did John Belushi.

Then, too, there are the many look-alike pills—caffeine pills made to look like pharmaceutical speed. They are sometimes sold to unwitting customers as the real deal.

Caffeine does tweak the neurons in a different manner than other addictive drugs, such as cocaine and heroin. In particular, it seems to have less of an effect on dopamine levels in the brain. Dopamine is a neurotransmitter associated with good feelings and is strongly associated with reinforcement and self-administration in addictive drugs. The most addictive drugs tend to increase concentrations of dopamine in the nucleus accumbens, a pleasure center in the middle of the brain.

But here, too, caffeine has some effect. In a 1997 literature review, Griffiths and Bridgette Garrett noted that caffeine does modestly enhance dopamine activity. This appears to be related to caffeine's effects on adenosine receptors, which are often adjacent to, and interact with, dopamine receptors. By blocking adenosine, caffeine amps up dopamine activity. And, they wrote, "Although more limited in scope, human studies also show that caffeine produces subjective, discriminative stimulus and reinforcing effects that have some similarities to those produced by cocaine and amphetamine."

For decades, some scientists have gone further than saying that caffeine causes addiction, arguing that the drug does little more than alleviate withdrawal symptoms for its habitual users. This would be analogous to a heroin addict taking a maintenance dose to avoid withdrawal. In 1930, the British drugs researcher W. E. Dixon, MD, wrote, "Knowledge of the action of caffeine on the mind of man has been obtained mainly by experiments on those who were already caffeine 'addicts,' and naturally enough on those people caffeine would be wholly beneficial."

A few scientists still say there is no net benefit to our caffeine jones but that we are simply a culture of twitchy caffeine addicts, stuck in a vicious circle of growing dose and tolerance.

In a 2005 literature review, researcher Jack James wrote, "Appropriately controlled studies show that the effects of caffeine on performance and mood, widely perceived to be net beneficial psychostimulant effects, are almost wholly attributable to reversal of adverse withdrawal effects associated with short periods of abstinence from the drug."

Griffiths believes that is an exaggerated perspective. And research continues to stack up against it. In research published in 2009, two scientists from Wake Forest School of Medicine tested whether caffeine has a greater effect in the withdrawal state compared with a normal caffeinated state. They found that caffeine had a greater effect after thirty hours of abstention, but improved attention and memory in both states. This supports the practice of regular caffeine users taking more caffeine than usual when facing an intellectually challenging task.

What all this means is that caffeine clearly has benefits, but they are offset to some degree for habitual users, because at least some of the effect goes toward simply alleviating withdrawal.

Some people, like Sally Satel, argue that coffee drinking, and caffeine use in general, is done more for secondary reasons—the flavor and the social interactions—than for the caffeine. Griffiths disagrees. He told me that caffeine drives patterns of consumption worldwide.

"You have the whole phenomenon of different cultures finding their own versions of caffeine. So if we were in Nigeria, we'd be chewing kola nuts. Tea in some countries, guarana in South America, yerba maté in South America," he said. "You have the majority of the world consuming it on a daily basis. And it's not about the taste of coffee, or soft drinks or tea, because you have it in different forms in different cultures, but it still drives the same habitual pattern of self-administration. The common denominator there is caffeine. And the studies that we and others have done have shown that it doesn't matter if it is delivered in coffee or soft drinks or capsules, it does the same thing, so it is clearly all about caffeine."

The varied preferences for different forms of caffeine in all corners of the globe suggest that it is the drug itself that is the object of our desire. Researchers have tested this by studying conditioned flavor preference.

In 1996, a British team reported on their research pairing capsules containing either one hundred milligrams of caffeine or a placebo with "novel-flavoured fruit juice" drinks. The subjects who were habitual caffeine users preferred the caffeine-paired drink. In essence, it was the subjects' fondness for caffeine that conditioned them to choose the caffeinated drink, not the flavor. "These results provide strong evidence for the existence of a reinforcing effect of caffeine, which probably plays a significant role in the acquisition of preferences for caffeine-containing drinks," they wrote.

One of Griffiths's more controversial papers emerged from a dis-agreement that started in the early 1980s between health advocates and the soft drink industry. Health advocates argued that caffeine was being used for its psychoactive effects. But the industry had long ar-gued that it added caffeine only to enhance the flavors of soft drinks. In a 1981 letter to the FDA contesting a proposal to tighten caffeine regulations, an attorney for Coca-Cola wrote, "The Coca-Cola Com-pany for decades has used caffeine as a component ingredient in Coca-Cola as a flavoring agent." In a 2008 report, the International Food Information Council stated, "Caffeine is added to soft drinks as a fla-voring agent; it imparts a bitterness that modifies the flavors of other components, both sour and sweet."

Griffiths and a colleague tested cola solutions with and without added caffeine to see if their twenty-five subjects could taste the differ-ence. At a caffeine concentration similar to Coca-Cola's, only two sub-jects were able to detect the caffeine flavor.

"The finding that only 8% of a group of regular cola soft drink consumers could detect the effect of the caffeine concentration found in most cola soft drinks is at variance with the claim made by soft drink manufacturers that caffeine is added to soft drinks because it plays an integral role in the flavor profile," Griffiths wrote. "It is valu-able for the general public, the medical community, and regulatory agencies to recognize that the high rates of consumption of caffeinated soft drinks more likely reflect the mood-altering and physical depen-dence producing effects of caffeine as a central nervous system-active drug than its subtle effects as flavoring agent."

Coca-Cola has not always downplayed caffeine's psychoactive ef-fects. Coke was originally marketed as a stimulant. But it has avoided talking about caffeine's kick for more than a century, since a landmark court case that we'll get to soon. And the soft drink industry is not alone in downplaying the role of an addictive drug in popular con-sumer products.

For more than a century, some of the most profitable companies in the United States have done their best to hook consumers on products that are addictive and deadly. The revelation that tobacco companies manipulated nicotine levels to maximize the addictive properties of cigarettes, and hid the health risks, was one of the biggest public health scandals of the twentieth century.

This is where the caffeine story gets particularly controversial. As he got further into his dedicated research on caffeine (which started out as a way to better understand other drugs of abuse), Griffiths began to see that the blending of caffeine into colas had striking similarities to the nicotine in cigarettes.

I asked him if it is a reach to make this analogy.

"No, not at all," he said.

"It's the same thing?"

"Absolutely," Griffiths said. "They are both centrally active psychoactive compounds and they both produce physical dependence and they both function as reinforcers and they are both intimately involved in the perpetuation of consumption of the product to which they are added."

In both cases, Griffiths believes it is important to have a conversation about the role drugs play in perpetuating habits.

"For a long time it was heresy to consider that cigarettes had anything to do with drugs," he said. "It was just a socially accepted habitual behavior that calmed the nerves or made people focus better."

He said the dialogue shifted with the recognition of the significant health risks associated with smoking. It was not the nicotine addiction, per se, that brought the issue to a head, but the health risks that came along with the addiction. As obesity rates have risen and smoking rates have declined, the former has replaced the latter as the greatest risk to public health in the United States. The link between obesity and sugary soft drinks is well established. In 2012, Harvard researchers writing in the *New England Journal of Medicine* had this to say: "During the past 30 years, the consumption of sugar-sweetened beverages has increased dramatically. Compelling evidence supports a

positive link between the consumption of sugar-sweetened beverages
and the risk of obesity; in the United States, both the intake of sugar-
sweetened beverages and the prevalence of obesity have more than
doubled since the late 1970s."

These obesity rates carry a hefty price tag in health care costs,
much of it funded by taxpayer dollars through Medicaid. One estimate
put the medical costs of obesity in the United States at $147 billion in
2008.

Kelly Brownell, an expert on food addiction and obesity, raised the
connection in an interview with *Yale Environment 360* magazine: "Caffeine, because it's so often coupled with calories, could become a real
player here, if you're consuming calories in something that has caffeine in it and the caffeine keeps you coming back for more because of
its mildly addictive nature then, again, you've got enough to create
real issues of health."

Coca-Cola has even acknowledged the obesity connection, if tacitly,
in an ad campaign launched in January 2013. Announcing the campaign in a press release, the corporation said, "A two-minute video,
titled 'Coming Together,' debuts tonight on national cable news. The
video encourages everyone to be mindful that all calories count in
managing your weight, including those in Coca-Cola products and in
all foods and beverages."

The nicotine-caffeine analogy might seem extreme, but the parallels are intriguing. It was not nicotine itself that constituted the primary health risk from cigarettes; it was the tar. So, too, with soft
drinks. It is not the caffeine that is the primary health risk, but the
sugar. In both cases, the delivery mechanisms (cigarettes and soda)
bundle the addictive drugs (nicotine and caffeine) with substances that
are deleterious to health (tar and sugar). And in both cases, the companies selling the products are well aware of the drugs' addictive qualities.

Griffiths is not the first to point out the similarities between caffeine and nicotine. Tobacco industry experts have often made the

same point, in order to trivialize nicotine's effects by comparing it to caffeine. In the 1990s, the University of Kentucky's Peter Rowell said, "I would say that nicotine is on the low end of the spectrum . . . more similar to caffeine than it is to the classical drugs of abuse in its pharmacological activity." John Robinson of R.J. Reynolds said, "I think the physiologic, pharmacologic, and behavioral effects of things like nicotine and caffeine are fundamentally different from addicting drugs like heroin and cocaine."

Crusading FDA commissioner David Kessler brought to a boiling point the issue of cigarette companies manipulating nicotine to addict customers. Consider his comments to a congressional subcommittee in March 1994: "The public thinks of cigarettes as simply blended tobacco rolled in paper. But they are much more than that. Some of today's cigarettes may, in fact, qualify as high technology nicotine delivery systems that deliver nicotine in precisely calculated quantities—quantities that are more than sufficient to create and to sustain addiction in the vast majority of individuals who smoke regularly."

Let's substitute "soft drinks" for "cigarettes" and "caffeine" for "nicotine," and see how it reads:

The public thinks of *soft drinks* as simply blended *beverages served in a can*. But they are much more than that. Some of today's *soft drinks* may, in fact, qualify as high technology *caffeine* delivery systems that deliver *caffeine* in precisely calculated quantities—quantities that are more than sufficient to create and to sustain addiction in the vast majority of individuals who *drink them* regularly.

Kessler went on to make this analogy: "Mr. Chairman, this kind of sophistication in setting levels of a physiologically active substance suggests that what we are seeing in the cigarette industry more and more resembles the actions of a pharmaceutical manufacturer."

Again, the analogy seems apt. For decades, Coca-Cola and all the other major soft drink bottlers have been using caffeine produced in pharmaceutical plants. Still, the beverage industry downplays the importance of caffeine's psychoactive effects.

The International Food Information Council Foundation, an industry-funded nonprofit, has posted a video clip on its Web site of Louisiana family practitioner Dr. Herbert Muncie glibly dismissing studies documenting caffeine withdrawal. People who reported withdrawal symptoms might have simply been "lethargic, headachy people before they took caffeine," he said.

The primary trade group, the American Beverage Association, made a dramatic claim in late 2011 in response to a report critical of the energy drink industry: "Furthermore, despite the suggestion in the report, caffeine is not a drug."

It was a claim that ran counter to a century of science. And it was disingenuous, because nobody on the planet understands caffeine better than the beverage industry. Even though per capita consumption of soft drinks peaked in the United States in 1998, and has declined since, Americans still lead the world in soda drinking. Carbonated soft drinks are worth $77 billion annually in the United States. The nation's top-selling soft drinks—Coke, Diet Coke, Pepsi, Mountain Dew, and Dr Pepper—have just one thing in common aside from carbonated water. They are all brewed with powdered caffeine.

Caffeine is so attractive that American bottlers blend more than ten million pounds of the addictive powder into their soft drinks every year. It is a tradition more than a century old, but still hidden in the shadows of American commerce.

PART II

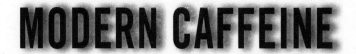

MODERN CAFFEINE

CHAPTER 6

The First Red Bull Was a Coke

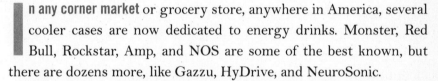

I n any corner market or grocery store, anywhere in America, several cooler cases are now dedicated to energy drinks. Monster, Red Bull, Rockstar, Amp, and NOS are some of the best known, but there are dozens more, like Gazzu, HyDrive, and NeuroSonic.

This is a relatively new phenomenon. Red Bull was only introduced in the United States in 1997, and the other drinks had yet to be formulated. It would seem natural to look at such a display and ask how canned, carbonated caffeine delivery mechanisms have changed so quickly. But the better question is this: What took so long?

To really understand energy drinks, we have to look back more than a century. In 1909, a man named Asa Candler was a dominant force in Atlanta. He owned a bank, warehouses full of cotton, and lots of real estate and had interests in railroads. In eight years he would become mayor of the fast-growing city.

Candler also owned Atlanta's tallest building, the seventeen-story Candler Building, which cast a long shadow over Peachtree Street. During its construction, he placed a bottle of Coca-Cola in the building's cornerstone. In the twenty years since he had wrested the rights to the Coca-Cola formula from its inventor, Candler had grown the business from a local novelty to a regional powerhouse. He was selling more than a million gallons of the drink annually: sixteen million servings. Having dominated the South, Candler was well on the way to conquering the entire United States beverage market. He dreamed of global distribution. Long before anyone had heard of energy drinks, Candler was making millions by hawking sweet drinks laced with caffeine.

Coke was marketed as a pick-me-up. It took its name from two stimulants that were part of its earliest formula: coca and kola, a caffeinated nut from Africa. A 1909 magazine ad shows a somewhat creepy, oversize hand extending from the doorway of a soda fountain, beckoning. "Tired?" the ad reads. "Come in and get a glass of Coca-Cola. It relieves fatigue." At that time, an eight-ounce serving of Coca-Cola contained eighty-one milligrams of caffeine, which is a pretty good dose. Less than a typical cup of coffee, but more than a strong cup of tea. A bit more than a SCAD. This is more than twice the amount of caffeine in a modern twelve-ounce can of Coca-Cola and nearly the exact amount contained in an eight-ounce can of Red Bull.

Put another way, the first Red Bull was a Coke.

But in 1909, Candler had a fight on his hands. His foe was Harvey Washington Wiley, a formidable opponent. As chairman of the U.S. Department of Agriculture's Bureau of Chemistry (which would eventually become the FDA) and its Interstate Pure Food Commission, he was charged with enforcing the Pure Food and Drugs Act.

Wiley had become famous for creating the Poison Squad in 1902. This was a group of twelve healthy men who ate foods treated with preservatives—including borax, formaldehyde, and saltpeter, among others—for several years, in order to understand their effects on human health. Journalists nicknamed Wiley "Old Borax" and the "crusading chemist," and the squad inspired this popular ditty: "Next week he'll give them mothballs à la Newburgh or else plain; Oh they may get over it but they'll never look the same." Wiley had used the publicity surrounding the Poison Squad to push through the Pure Food and Drugs Act in 1906.

Candler was worried because after Wiley had alerted Americans to the dangers of preservatives, he set his sights on caffeine, stating that it was an addictive poison and should not be marketed to children. Interestingly, Wiley was not going after coffee, which he drank daily, but rather the caffeine that was a key ingredient in Coca-Cola. He said the beverage did not contain two items its name suggested—coca and kola—and did contain one he considered as addictive as opium and marijuana: caffeine.

Their showdown began on October 20, 1909, in East Ridge, Tennessee, where federal agents waited for a freight truck approaching from Georgia. When the truck crossed the state line, the load became interstate commerce, and thus the jurisdiction of the United States government. The agents seized the load: forty barrels and twenty kegs of cola syrup, en route from Coca-Cola's main plant in Atlanta to a bottling plant in Chattanooga. They charged the Coca-Cola Company with violating the Pure Food and Drugs Act by adulterating their beverage with a harmful ingredient: caffeine.

The *Atlanta Constitution* ran a brief item, the first trickle in what would soon be barrels of ink spilled on the story:

> Chattanooga, Tenn., October 23—An information has been filed by United States District Attorney Penland libeling a carload of coca-cola sirup shipped from the Coca-Cola Company at Atlanta, to the Coca-Cola Bottling Works of Chattanooga. The grounds for the libel, as set out in the information, are that coca-cola contains caffeine, which, the information alleges, is a substance deleterious to health. The information further alleges that the consignment libeled is misbranded in that it does not contain the active principal of cocoa [coca] leaves, as the government claims is indicated by the brand on the barrels, and that the caffeine it contains is extracted from tea leaves and not from the coca [kola] nut.

This showdown between the U.S. government and Coca-Cola was more than a historical curiosity. It also set the trajectory for a century of caffeine regulation.

It took two years for the case to come to trial. Finally, in March 1911, Harvey Washington Wiley traveled from his home in Washington, D.C., to Chattanooga to watch the trial, by then known as *United States v. Forty Barrels and Twenty Kegs of Coca-Cola*, or simply "the famous Coca-Cola trial."

Things looked bad to Wiley from the start. He checked into the elegant Hotel Patten, then learned it was owned by J. T. Lupton, the Coca-Cola bottler in Chattanooga. "I proposed to bring the action in the District of Columbia, where our experts were readily accessible, but Solicitor McCabe ordered the suit brought in Chattanooga, where the great bottling works of the company were located and where the sentiment would he heavily in favor of the company," Wiley wrote. "I went down there and found that the very hotel where I was to stay was owned by the Coca Cola people. There could not have been a more favorable place for the defense except Atlanta."

After a week of testimony, the government rested its case on March 21, its lawyers feeling they had made a strong showing against Coca-Cola. The government's best-known food expert was silent throughout the proceedings. Wiley sat through the entire trial, but felt it would be inappropriate to testify because he had not personally conducted caffeine research. It was a decision he later rued.

The jury heard testimony from Dr. Louis Schaefer, of the Schaefer Alkaloid Works in Lakewood, New Jersey. Schaefer's company produced the key Coca-Cola ingredient known as Merchandise No. 5. He testified that he produced it using "decocanized" coca leaves and powdered kola nuts. Others testified about the caffeine content of coffee and chocolate purchased in Atlanta, for comparison.

But much of the testimony was anecdotal and biased. Testifying for Coca-Cola, Chattanooga physician B. H. Brown spoke about assessing the drink's effects on people. According to the *Atlanta Constitution*,

"Dr. Brown testified that he had examined 100 men of an average age of 24 years, all picked by the coca-cola people, and found none who had been affected by the use of coca-cola."

And some of the testimony was remarkably unprofessional. One of Coca-Cola's experts, Dr. R. C. Witthaus, took the stand to state that caffeine was not a poison. Federal attorneys then presented Witthaus with a book he had written, in which he not only declared caffeine a poison, but he cited thirteen fatal cases of overdose. Philadelphia pharmacologist Horatio Wood was also caught up by the government attorneys, after his own written works on caffeine as a muscle poison contradicted his testimony. (In both cases, the witnesses asserted that they had copied the contradicting parts of their books from other sources, and those passages therefore were likely inaccurate.)

So the trial was strong on emotion, anecdotal evidence, and pseudoscience, which is not surprising for an important court case of that era. What *is* surprising is what came next.

Coca-Cola had some momentum entering the third week of the trial, and its lawyers were about to pull out their secret weapon. A few months earlier, the company's legal team happened onto a gap in their defense, realizing that nearly all caffeine research to date had been conducted on animals. Coca-Cola needed to find someone to conduct research on humans—to counter Wiley's assertion that Coca-Cola led to mental deficiency—and quickly.

A few years earlier, the researcher W. H. R. Rivers had conducted a study that concluded that caffeine lessened fatigue and increased the capacity for work. But the only subjects were Rivers and another man.

After more established psychologists turned down Coca-Cola's offer, for fear of sullying their reputations by doing the bidding of a large business, Harry Levi Hollingworth took on the contract. He had recently earned a PhD from Columbia University and was teaching at its Barnard College.

Time was tight, and Hollingworth had his day job to do. His wife, Leta Hollingworth, and a pool of assistants did most of the day-to-day work. In just forty days, they rented a Manhattan apartment, mustered sixteen subjects—including abstainers and occasional, moderate, and regular caffeine users—and administered an elegant series of tests. The researchers evaluated cognition, sensory abilities, and motor skills under conditions of caffeine abstinence and moderate and heavy use. They conducted blind and double-blind experiments, using caffeine capsules and placebos as well as Coca-Cola syrup with and without caffeine.

The Hollingworths wrapped up the research shortly after the trial began in Chattanooga. Harry Hollingworth testified on March 27, confident in his comprehensive studies. The next day, the *Daily Times of Chattanooga* reported, "Dr. Hollingsworth's [*sic*] testimony consumed a greater part of the morning hearing. He produced various charts and scientific apparatus to substantiate his belief that caffeine had no secondary depression. His testimony was by far the most interesting and technical of any yet introduced. Cross-examination failed to shake any of his deductions."

Despite the fact that things were looking up, the Coca-Cola attorneys did not want to take their chances with a jury. A week after Hollingworth's testimony, they introduced a motion to dismiss, claiming the caffeine they blended into the product was an ingredient inherent to their recipe, that Coca-Cola would not be Coca-Cola without the caffeine.

Judge Edward Sanford agreed. In his ruling he wrote, "The caffeine contained in the article Coca-Cola is one of its regular, habitual and essential constituents, and that without its presence, that is, if it were de-caffeinized, so to speak, the product would lack one of its essential elements and fail to produce upon the consumer a characteristic if not the most characteristic effect which is obtained from its use."

It seems notable that the judge highlighted the caffeine kick as perhaps the most characteristic effect of the drink, but this was before Coca-Cola rebranded caffeine as a mere flavoring agent.

Judge Sanford went one step further and suggested the company could not very well sell its product without the caffeine: "In short, Coca-Cola without caffeine would not be 'Coca-Cola' as it is known to the public and would not produce the effect which the Coca-Cola bought by the public under that name produces, and if it were sold as 'Coca-Cola' without containing caffeine the public buying it under this name would be in fact deceived."

Coca-Cola and Hollingworth won the battle, but the war continued.

One of the faults of the Pure Food and Drugs Act was its lack of specificity (and length: it was just six pages long). In 1912, Congress was considering amendments to make the law easier to interpret and enforce, including one that would have added caffeine to a list of substances considered habit forming or deleterious.

At a hearing on the amendments before the House Committee on Interstate and Foreign Commerce, Wiley revived his concerns about Coca-Cola. (He appeared before the committee as a private citizen, having resigned a month earlier, following a series of contentious, highly politicized, and personal challenges to his work.)

Wiley mentioned a letter he had recently received from a Kentucky physician concerned about the Coca-Cola habit. "I am noticing with regret the way it is getting a hold on people," Dr. O. C. Robertson wrote Wiley. "In my practice I notice that the regular drinkers of Coca-Cola are developing chronic digestive troubles, and all of them will lie about drinking to excess; they appear to take on the characteristics of a morphine patient."

But Wiley was quickly interrupted by Congressman Edward Hamilton, who noted that "the amount of caffeine in the ordinary glass of Coca-Cola would not exceed the amount of caffeine in an ordinary cup of coffee. . . . And that it would be no more a habit-forming drug on that account than the habit of drinking coffee, and that would never be considered a habit-forming drug."

The committee members worried that adding caffeine to the list in the amendment would mean establishing that it is a habit-forming drug. So Hamilton asked the obvious question: "What will we do with coffee? I speak now with very superficial knowledge, in fact, no knowledge at all, but apparently it would be as injurious to the human system if persisted in as coca cola."

Wiley responded, "Apparently, yes. In point of fact I do not think it is as much because coffee is taken with our meals, and Coca-Cola is a drug that is poured into an empty stomach as a rule. Caffeine has a more vigorous action under these circumstances, and we all know how we keep our children from drinking coffee and tea, and how we ourselves would not drink strong coffee—at least, I would not—just before going to bed. I would toss all night in my bed."

Gaining a full head of steam, Wiley let loose a blistering tirade: "Why should the people of this country be subjected to this awful drugging? Why should your fatigue be relieved and thus wear you out all the more because you don't know you are tired? Fatigue is nature's signal that there is danger ahead. Will you make a railroad more safe if you go along and take all the red lights away from the open switches? They are the marks of danger. What is fatigue? It is nature's notices that you have done enough. You take a glass of Coca-Cola. You see it on every sign. 'Relieves Fatigue.' How does it relieve fatigue—by furnishing any more energy or food? No: but by taking away the sense of feeling—striking out the sense of danger. When you are tired, you ought to rest, and not drink Coca-Cola."

Wiley insisted that the law would not apply to coffee and tea, because caffeine was not an additive but a natural constituent in those cases. He was earnest and adamant, but showed a sense of humor by taking a jab at restaurants that served weak coffee. Asked if a bottle of Coca-Cola had the same amount of caffeine as a cup of coffee, he replied, "The same volume. The volume of a cup will carry about as much as a cup of coffee. Coffee varies, though. Some restaurants you go into you do not get much caffeine. [Laughter.]"

Coca-Cola attorney Harold Hirsch said the issue should not be determined by Congress while the matter was working its way through the courts, via the appeal of the Forty Barrels case. Summing up for Coca-Cola, Hirsch noted that Wiley had failed to testify when he had a chance in the courtroom in Chattanooga. And he said the trial had made several things clear: "That the scientific evidence produced shows that caffeine is not habit forming or deleterious. That the evidence adduced at Chattanooga shows that the extravagant statements made in regard to Coca-Cola are not true. That Coca-Cola comes under the same category as coffee and tea."

Caffeine stayed off the list.

⚡

Wiley landed on his feet after leaving his government post. He went to work running an experimental lab for *Good Housekeeping* magazine, eventually developing the Good Housekeeping Seal of approval. He also used its pages to keep up a drumbeat of Coca-Cola criticism.

The U.S. government appealed the Forty Barrels ruling and pursued the case for another five years. In 1916, the case reached the U.S. Supreme Court, which remanded it to the district court. But the lower court never reached a decision. Coca-Cola changed its formula in the interim, and argued that the original case no longer applied. In 1917, the court agreed. As part of a consent decree, Coca-Cola did not admit to the charges of misbranding or adulteration, and it did get its syrup back (though it is hard to imagine what it did with the eight-year-old stuff), but had to pay the court costs.

Coca-Cola did reduce the caffeine in its formula as an outcome of the trial (though there seems to be no written documentation quantifying this). Caffeine concentrations have varied in the years since, but Coca-Cola's current formulation of thirty-four milligrams of caffeine per twelve-ounce serving was certainly well established by 1958, when Coca-Cola argued to the FDA that its current formula had been in "common use for such a long period of time."

⚡

The case raised but failed to resolve the questions regulators, scientists, and consumers are still considering today: How much caffeine is too much? Is it different when added to soft drinks as opposed to naturally occurring in coffee or tea? Is it habit forming? Should it be marketed to youths? How should the federal government regulate it?

The trial presaged a century of ambivalence toward caffeine. On one hand, Americans' fierce cravings have made colas, teas, coffee, and energy drinks exceedingly popular. On the other, many of us are beset with nagging suspicions that caffeine may indeed be an addictive poison.

It is a situation of cognitive dissonance, again best exemplified by Wiley. In November 1912, he gave a talk to the National Coffee Association at New York's Hotel Astor. Although his talk was titled "The Advantages of Coffee as America's National Beverage," the crusading chemist could not resist poking a stick at his hosts. The *New York Times* quoted Wiley as saying, "Assuming that the moderate use of coffee is not harmful, yet I am a moderate drinker and I can lose a night's sleep by taking one extra cup of coffee, and a small cup at that. It is your duty to warn people of the dangers of overindulgence."

Still, Wiley conceded that he was like most Americans and drank coffee every day. "'I know it does me no good,' he said, 'but I like it.'"

The Hollingworths did well by the Coca-Cola contract. Leta soon earned a PhD from Columbia and became a pioneering feminist psychologist, and Harry later served as president of the American Psychological Association.

Hollingworth compiled his research, which was so authoritative that it is still referenced today, in a 1912 book, *The Influence of Caffein on Mental and Motor Efficiency*. The comments of his subjects provide familiar insights into the caffeinated state. One, an abstainer before the trial, was administered four grains of caffeine (about the equivalent of a twelve-ounce cup of strong coffee) and had this reaction: "Gradual rise of spirits till 4:00. Then a period of exuberance, of good feeling. Fanciful ideas rampant. Had three sudden attacks of perspiration. Gradual decrease of exhilaration but continued sensations such as felt after shock. Trembling of knees and hands. Uncertainty as to truth of ideas, so feel cautious." Another, a regular user before the trial, wrote this on a caffeine-free day: "Felt like a 'bone head' all day. My head was dull more than usual. Otherwise all right."

In a test on mathematical calculations, Hollingworth noted, "All squads reveal a most pronounced stimulation following caffein. This stimulation amounts to a considerable per cent. . . . No evidence of any secondary depression is found."

Like all good science, Hollingworth's caffeine studies raised more questions than they answered. Hollingworth wrote, "It must be said that our present knowledge concerning the precise mode of action of drugs on nervous tissue is very inadequate. That the increased capacity for work is produced is clearly demonstrated. That this result is a genuine drug effect . . . the carefully controlled tests here reported prove beyond any doubt. But whether this increased capacity comes from a new supply of energy introduced or rendered available by the drug action, or whether energy already available comes to be employed more effectively, or whether the inhibition of secondary afferent impulses is eliminated, or whether fatigue sensations are weakened and the individual's standard of performance thereby raised, no one seems to know." These are questions scientists have wrestled with for a century.

A 1912 editorial in *The Journal of the American Medical Association* welcomed the research. "It is gratifying to have the effects on the human system of a drug like caffeine so investigated by rigorous scientific tests at the hands of capable investigators; only in this way will there be provided an adequate basis for correct conclusions as to the possible dangers of the use of caffeine-containing beverages."

Hollingworth did more than quantify caffeine's benefits; he also set an enduring standard for methods of studying applied psychology. And his general observations about how caffeine affects the body and brain still hold up today, though they have been refined by modern researchers.

Aside from generating weeks' worth of headlines, the famous Chattanooga trial had three lasting impacts. It prompted the Hollingworths' pioneering research on caffeine's effects on human physiology. It framed the basic questions about regulating caffeine that remain today. But mostly it cleared the way for caffeinated soft drinks to continue marching across the country.

CHAPTER 7

Hot Caffeine

⚡

Coca-Cola did not get its zest from its namesake ingredients cocaine and kola, but from the powdered caffeine Candler blended into the drink. While coca and cola sound more exotic than caffeine, the latter was doing the heavy lifting.

In 1905, a small chemical company in St. Louis began producing caffeine for Coca-Cola. It was the third product for the fledgling company, which was already producing vanillin and saccharine for the beverage company. For decades afterward, the company refined caffeine from waste tea leaves to supply the soft drink industry. The company was Monsanto.

Monsanto eventually grew into a massive worldwide corporation, best known for producing pesticides like Roundup as well as corn that is genetically modified to resist those same pesticides. But it owes its early success to caffeine, which Monsanto chemist Gaston DuBois credited with "keeping us solvent for 10 years" in the early 1900s.

As demand increased, other companies began extracting caffeine from tea leaves. In 1918, the periodical *Drug and Chemical Markets* reported on a new chemical company in Formosa (now known as Taiwan). Its factory planned to produce five thousand pounds of caffeine annually, to be refined in Tokyo. The article noted, "The amount of caffeine which can be extracted from Taiwan tea varies from 3 to 10 pounds per 1,000 pounds of raw material according to the quality of the tea used."

By 1921, Monsanto's Levi Cooke was asking Congress for tariffs protecting against imported caffeine. "It requires fifty pounds of tea waste to manufacture one pound of caffeine, and, of course, all the tea waste is imported," Cooke testified. He asked Congress to either decrease the duty on tea waste or increase the duty on finished caffeine, to give domestic production a competitive edge over Japanese caffeine.

"The Monsanto Chemical Works consider it mandatory that there be a clear protection of at least one dollar per pound on the finished caffeine, in order that its plant for the production of this article can continue in operation," Cooke said. "Such caffeine as is imported, and it will continue to be imported, will thus pay a revenue and competitive conditions being preserved in the United States will prevent a Japanese monopoly from being created on this important article." Soon, a Brazilian company was also in the game, processing more than 13,000 pounds of maté daily to make about 132 pounds of caffeine.

As soft drinks evolved from oddball patent medicines into America's beloved beverages, the demand for caffeine increased. The bitter white powder became a commodity, and a competitive international industry was scrambling to meet the bottlers' ever-growing demands.

By 1945, four firms were producing caffeine in the United States. Two Maywood, New Jersey, companies and Monsanto were extracting caffeine from tea (Monsanto was also extracting theobromine from cocoa residues in Virginia and shipping them to Montreal to be processed into caffeine), and one company, General Foods Corporation, was extracting caffeine from coffee, as part of the process of making decaf. They still do it that way in Texas.

⚡

A couple of miles east of the cluster of skyscrapers that marks downtown Houston, on the rail line extending to the oil refineries at the port, sits a sprawling industrial building with pipes and ducts winding along the roof. The whole complex smells of roasting coffee. When the wind blows right, you can smell it wafting through downtown Houston.

This is the Maximus Coffee Group plant. It is massive, the size of nine Walmarts. It's so large, in fact, that Leo Vasquez, the executive vice president, had to ask directions as he led me to the southwestern corner of the plant.

En route, we passed coffee being roasted, ground, and packaged every which way. It was mesmerizing to watch the jars and bags whip off the line—a cacophony of clinking, swooshing, and thunking as coffee flowed into vacuum-packed bricks, pods, jars, and even tea bags. Another part of the building held the instant coffee plant, where coffee is brewed, as in a giant percolator, and then sprayed into a hot blast of air and instantly dried into a powder.

Square, white "super sacks" sat here and there in the warehouse, each holding two thousand pounds of coffee. A truck backed in to a loading bay, tipped up, and dumped a twenty-foot container full of coffee into a hopper. Vasquez said the Maximus coffees go all over the world: to Indonesia, Taiwan, and Eastern Europe. They employ four hundred people, and parts of the plant run 24-7.

Once a Ford factory, the large plant eventually became a Maxwell House coffee roaster. Its red neon sign—reading MAXWELL HOUSE and showing coffee dripping from a tilted coffee cup—adorned the tall tower at the front of the plant and became a Houston landmark. The sign came down when Maximus bought the coffee plant from Kraft in 2007. The plant is a blend of high-tech and low—new roasting and packing machines on the production lines, all linked up by aging concrete corridors and steel stairs.

Vasquez took me to a dimly lit control room, where three men sat inside a circular cockpit watching thirteen large-screen monitors. It looked like a miniature NASA mission control room, but here the men were conducting another sort of high-tech operation. They were decaffeinating coffee.

It is an involved process, originally developed by the German company Café Hag (now owned by Kraft Foods). First, the men moisturize the green (unroasted) coffee beans. They come in at 12 percent moisture and are sprayed with steam and hot water to bring them up to 35 percent. The coffee beans are then pneumatically blown to the top of a 280-foot tower with two parallel sides, each including several large chambers. The walls of the chambers are six inches thick, clad on the inside with stainless steel. Each of the valves between the chambers weighs as much as a Volkswagen.

The beans flow back down through the chambers while carbon dioxide is pumped through the beans from the bottom up. It is not just any carbon dioxide; it is supercritical carbon dioxide, so hot and under so much pressure—more than 3,500 p.s.i., and 190 degrees Fahrenheit—that it behaves more like a liquid than like a gas. This allows it to pass through the beans like a ghost, performing a neat bit of alchemy—stripping away the caffeine while leaving the coffee flavor intact.

Looking over the control room, Vasquez told me that nobody produces more decaf without chemicals than Maximus. The plant cost more than $100 million when it was built in the 1980s. Because it would be unimaginably expensive to make another such plant today, Vasquez said infrastructure cost is a "significant barrier to entry" for any potential competitors.

In the control room, Bo Wheatley, who oversees the decaffeination process, described the last step. After it flows up through the beans, the caffeine-laden carbon dioxide is blended into a column of water. Routed into a chamber where the pressure drops, the caffeine and water separate from the carbon dioxide, which is recovered for reuse. Gesturing to a scale model of the decaffeination vessels, Wheatley said, "Right here is where the caffeine decides, 'I like the water more than the CO_2, so I am going to stay with the water.'"

The coffee, sans caffeine, flows out of the bottom of the tower, forty-five hundred pounds every forty-five minutes. The process is constant. Maximus decaffeinates more than one hundred million pounds of coffee beans annually.

The water, which has a weak concentration of caffeine of about one quarter of a percent, flows into two 20,000-gallon tanks out back. The tanks are labeled on the sides: HOT CAFFEINE. From there, it goes through two concentrators, where steam coils heat the solution to evaporate the water, leaving a highly concentrated liquid. Finally, the brew flows into an arch-topped dryer about the size of a small wood-shed.

⚡

Vasquez opened a hatch in the dryer's stainless steel steam hood and showed me where the concentrated brownish liquid—looking like light brown chocolate syrup—poured onto a hot rotating drum. The water steamed quickly away, leaving a flaky powder residue, which was then scraped off by a blade as the cylinder rotated. The powder was tan—the color of café con leche, mid-Atlantic sand, Colorado River mud. "That's the caffeine," said Vasquez. The powder flowed down through a hatch and poured into a plastic-lined cardboard box sitting on a pallet on the floor below. We went downstairs to have a look, and Vasquez lifted the plastic hood covering the top so we could watch it streaming in. The box held one thousand pounds of crude caffeine, which was about 95 percent pure (it still contained about 3 percent water and 2 percent impurities and would need further refining before being sold as caffeine).

"What we produce here is a naturally generated caffeine. And you can get a bunch of it at once," said Vasquez. "There's no shortage of demand for naturally processed, chemical-free caffeine."

Elsewhere in the plant, Vasquez showed me a spick-and-span room that looked like a biology lab with slate counters and deep sinks, full of beakers, flasks, pipettes, and vials. On one end of the room was a tasting area. On the other end, a small machine sat on a long work counter. It was a caffeine-counting machine. This is the lab where technicians ensure that the coffee qualifies as decaf.

Ruben Cerda, who runs the lab, said the machine is a "high-pressure liquid chromatography," or HLPC, device. Cerda and his lab assistants use ten-microliter samples in little vials to test the decaf they are producing. Any coffee with less than 0.3 percent caffeine is considered decaf, and Cerda said most of their samples come in at 0.25 percent.

For comparison, he says, most Colombian coffees will have between 1.2 and 1.9 percent caffeine. Other arabicas are often slightly higher, between 1.4 percent and 2.1 percent caffeine. And those caffeine-rich robustas? Cerda said they often have 2.6 percent caffeine.

Bruce Goldberger and his colleagues found that a typical sixteen-ounce cup of decaf contains ten to fourteen milligrams of caffeine (about one-fifth of a SCAD). It's not much caffeine, but a couple of cups can certainly deliver a small kick, especially to people who are caffeine sensitive.

⚡

Leaving the plant, we passed more thousand-pound boxes of caffeine lined up near a loading dock. Maximus sends the caffeine to Mexico to be refined in the hills above Veracruz. At forty boxes per shipment, the company ships more than a million pounds of crude caffeine annually. Since no company refines caffeine in the United States, all of the finished product, known as "caffeine anhydrous," is imported. Once refined, most of the caffeine will be sold to soft drink bottlers.

A million pounds sounds like a lot of caffeine powder, but it is just a drop in the bucket. Pepsi requires about 1.2 million pounds just to blend into the Mountain Dew it sells in the United States annually. Energy drinks are the most conspicuous consumers of powdered caffeine, but in 2010, Monster, Red Bull, and Rockstar, combined, used less caffeine powder than Mountain Dew alone; Mountain Dew's caffeine concentration is lower, but its sales are much higher. Coke and Diet Coke, the nation's top two soda brands, require another 3.5 million pounds.

In 1975, soft drinks passed coffee as America's favorite caffeinated beverage and never looked back. Soft drink sales have been led by Coca-Cola, the company Asa Candler built. The Atlanta corporation now has the world's best-known brand, and powdered caffeine is the key attraction.

Eight of the nation's top ten soft drinks are made with caffeine powder. Some are cola flavored, others are citrus flavored; some have sugar, some do not. Aside from carbonated water, caffeine is the only common denominator.

To meet the needs of bottlers like Coca-Cola, Pepsi, and Dr Pepper Snapple, Americans import more than fifteen million pounds of powdered caffeine annually. That's enough to fill three hundred 40-foot shipping containers. Imagine a freight train two miles long, each car loaded to the brim with psychoactive powder.

After touring the plant, I stopped to meet Maximus president Carlos de Aldecoa Bueno. The third-generation coffee trader's office sits in the northwest corner of the building, with a view toward the Houston skyline.

His grandfather started a coffee business in Spain, then moved it to Veracruz, Mexico. His father then moved the business to the Houston area and still runs another, methylene chloride–based, decaffeination plant nearby. De Aldecoa started out warehousing coffee, and then assumed control of the Maxwell House plant when Kraft wanted to get out from under the operation.

De Aldecoa was clear that his primary products are coffee and decaf coffee. Caffeine is just a by-product to him, and one the company nearly stopped processing when cheap caffeine from China first flooded the market.

But he said the market has improved, and his caffeine is selling at a premium. "Everyone is going to natural products overall," he said. "A few companies call it out as natural caffeine. It's a good by-product, as opposed to the synthetic caffeine coming out of China."

Up until the 1950s, powdered caffeine was typically made the old-fashioned way, by extracting it from coffee, tea, guarana, or kola nuts. That is the way Monsanto began producing caffeine in 1905. And that is the way they still do it at Maximus.

But by the World War II years, demand was outstripping capacity. In a 1942 War Production Board memo, John Smiley, chief of the Beverage and Tobacco Branch, emphasized the importance of soft drinks to morale. He wrote, "Soft drinks are an inseparable part of our way of life, and it is the desire of the highest authority in the land that the people be not prevented from having their soft drinks."

But Smiley said caffeine supplies were imperiled. "A careful study . . . reveals the fact that caffeine manufacturers are literally 'scraping the bin' as their supplies of caffeine bearing raw materials are about to reach the vanishing point," he wrote. "Stocks of caffeine in the hands of soft drink bottlers are also dwindling away and it is only a matter of a month or two before their supplies will be entirely exhausted."

This turned out to be more important than a temporary crimp in the supply chain. Robert Woodruff, the master marketer who led Coca-Cola for decades, saw soldiers as consumers who were critical to his growth strategy. According to Mark Pendergrast in his history of Coca-Cola, Woodruff proclaimed that every soldier should get a bottle of Coca-Cola for five cents, no matter where he was. Soldiers chugged ten billion Cokes during the war and became the loyal customers who helped colas knock coffee from its pedestal.

Coke, Pepsi, Dr Pepper, and Royal Crown all reduced their caffeine content by an average of 54 percent during the war years, but supplies were still tight. In 1945, annual caffeine production totaled a million pounds. "Tea wastes are [the] largest single source in domestic solvent extraction processes, and far more important than coffee which provides the chemical through decaffeination," *Chemical and Engineering News* reported. "A practical process for the production of caffeine by complete synthesis would probably displace foreign sources for theobromine and caffeine in this country. . . . Wholly synthesized caffeine," the journal reported, cost twice as much as extracted caffeine, which then sold for less than three dollars per pound.

Later that year, the same journal reported that an American firm was taking up the challenge, by diversifying from its tradition of producing natural caffeine: "Monsanto Chemical Co. has disclosed its intention to free the United States from dependency on foreign-produced natural sources of caffeine through construction and operation of what will be the world's first large-scale plant for the manufacture of synthetic caffeine."

Caffeine synthesis, assembling the chemical from its building blocks instead of carving it away from plant material, was a German innovation. The chemist Emil Fischer pioneered the process in 1895, using uric acid as the primary building block. (This was one of the achievements that earned him a Nobel Prize in 1902.)

And it turned out that Germans had also pioneered the industrial production of synthetic caffeine, a few years ahead of Monsanto. The German company Boehringer Ingelheim had built a large synthetic caffeine plant in 1942, though Americans may not have been aware of it. Then, as now, all of the major caffeine-consuming nations in Europe and North America lacked any commercially viable caffeinated crop. Chocolate, coffee, and tea are imported from less developed countries to sate our appetites for legal stimulants. It can be challenging to keep the supply lines open, even in peacetime, but the war years were especially fraught, on both sides of the Atlantic.

Pfizer was not far behind Monsanto in switching caffeine sources. In 1947, the pharmaceutical company bought a New Jersey plant that extracted caffeine from tea leaves. It soon shut down that operation and consolidated its caffeine production in Groton, Connecticut, where it made synthetic caffeine. In 1953, Pfizer touted its product in a full-page ad in the trade journal *American Bottler*: "Pfizer, with its large modern plant at Groton, Conn., is now one of the world's largest basic producers of Caffeine."

Despite shifting its production to synthetic caffeine, by 1957, Monsanto was under ever-growing pressure from cheap, imported caffeine. *Chemical and Engineering News* reported that Monsanto had lowered prices from $3.00 per pound to $2.50, the lowest price since 1940, to try to compete with overseas producers.

The Pfizer plant mostly stayed out of the news for decades, but on June 20, 1995, residents of Groton, Connecticut, noticed a yellow cloud rising above the plant on the Thames River. Under the headline WORKERS EVACUATED AT CAFFEINE UNIT, the *New London Day* ran the story the next day: "About 100 workers at Pfizer, Inc. were evacuated Tuesday after a cloud of nitrogen oxide was released from a chemical manufacturing building at the plant. . . . The gas was released about 1:15 p.m. in a building used to produce caffeine, company spokeswoman Kate Robbins said. . . . The caffeine building has been closed off until investigators determine the cause of the release, Robbins said."

But despite the presence of a "caffeine building" at a pharmaceutical plant in Connecticut, most Americans remained unaware that a key constituent in the country's favorite beverage was often chemically synthesized.

I wanted to learn about caffeine synthesis and to see the process. But I found out that the Pfizer plant was long gone, and nobody was synthesizing caffeine in the United States any longer. The caffeine industry had been offshored.

CHAPTER 8

China White

Shijiazhuang (sure-DIA-JUON) is a city with so few tourist attractions that neither of my thick China guidebooks—thirteen hundred pages in all—even mentions it. The capital of Hebei province, it is already a city of ten million and growing like wildfire. It is larger than any city in the United States, but most Americans know nothing about it. It is also home to the many pharmaceutical companies that have factories in the surrounding towns.

To find the pharmaceutical plant I wanted to see, I had to take a taxi about thirty kilometers southwest on Luan Chen, a rough concrete road where tractors hauled trailers full of rebar, mothers carried daughters on rear bicycle racks, and black Mercedes and Audi sedans, and even Porches, vied for space with taxis and buses. Along the way we passed dozens of skyscrapers under construction. But not clustered tightly, as in Manhattan; rather two here, five there, three groups of three, just sort of scattered about the landscape and fading into the brown pall. The air was nearly opaque, the sun's light dimmed at noon by the pollution. The road disappeared into the distance.

Finally, the road passed into an older village of one-, two-, and three-story houses and apartments. We took a right on Fuqiang Road, a dusty, quiet road with a couple of storefronts and sidewalk vendors deep-frying food. But soon the frying aromas gave way to the unmistakable sour smell of chemicals.

At first, it was faint, the scent you notice in the garden aisle at the hardware store. But it got stronger as we approached a smallish power plant with tall brick smokestacks, tucked in among the acres of factories that have grown up beside the village.

Winding away from the power plant, like the legs of a slender squid, pipes carried steam to a half dozen chemical plants. The pipes crossed over the road, traveled down the sidewalks on failing metal stanchions, the pipe insulation unraveling in spots, and disappeared over the six-foot cement walls that lined the road. By now the chemical smell was acrid.

Then, off to the left, a vision from a dystopian future: an abandoned chemical plant, shuttered so suddenly that a chair still sat before a desk at the guardhouse just inside the gate, with a clipboard unfurled to a certain page, awaiting someone to check something off. But *shuttered* is not the right word, for half the windows were smashed, and rags streamed out. Bags of stockpiled chemicals sat inside the broken first-floor windows. The place reeked—a chemical stench to make you gag—and a tall rusty tank leaked a tarry sludge.

Another three hundred meters along, past the veterinary medicine plant and just before the amino acid factory, was a tidier facility with four buses at the curb and seventy-five or so bikes and electric scooters parked on the sidewalk. Beyond the guardhouse and the blue and white administrative building I glimpsed what looked like a mini oil refinery—a complex network of pipes snaking between tanks.

That's where I caught a waft of a strong but slightly different smell. The odor of cat pee. Ammonia.

This is the world's largest caffeine factory. This modest chemical plant, run by CSPC Innovation Pharmaceutical Company, shipped 4.7 million pounds of caffeine to the United States in 2011. If you drink any soda at all, or any of the hundreds of new caffeinated energy prod-

ucts, you've likely consumed some caffeine produced here, outside Shijiazhuang.

This CSPC plant, along with two others in China—Shandong Xin-
hua and Tianjin Zhongan—and India's Kudos Chemie, synthesize
more than half of all the caffeine we consume in the United States. All
of these plants declined requests for site tours, and Coke and Pepsi,
the world's top two powdered caffeine consumers, would not arrange
a visit to any caffeine production facility. I tried to make connections
with manufacturers in three countries through their corporate offices,
customers, middlemen, flavoring houses, academics, journalists, and
diplomats. It wasn't terribly surprising that the companies turned me
away—pharmaceutical plants often arrange tours for customers but
have little incentive to allow journalists to visit. But the more rejec-
tions I got, the more determined I became.

BASF, the German company with the longest history in producing
synthetic caffeine and the world's largest chemical company, flatly denied my request. Kudos Chemie, which has quickly become a major
supplier to U.S. bottlers, considered it, then responded with this e-
mail:

> Dear Mr. Carpenter,
>
> Please refer to the subject matter, the undersign had
> discussed the issue with higher authorities of our
> organization, the management <u>does not agree</u> for viewing
> the process of Caffeine manufacturing & other details.
> This is the fundamental policy/charter of Company.
>
> Kindly excuse us, . . .

The underlined and bolded phrase "does not agree" seemed to cap-
ture all of my frustration. Still, I decided to visit China, where two
plants had only provided vague answers to my inquiries—they had
not agreed to let me visit, but had not given me a flat-out no. Of the
two, CSPC was the largest and most intriguing. I told CSPC that I

would be coming to Shijiazhuang and that I looked forward to visiting the plant. After months of badgering, CSPC finally denied my request for a tour at one thirty a.m. on the day I was leaving Beijing for Shijiazhuang.

The e-mail I received looked like this: 您好！由于您是外籍采访人士 经我们咨询市委市政府相关部门 接受任何外方采访发言均需要官方批准 所以暂不能满足您的要求！不便之处 还请您另做安排！很遗憾！

The exclamation points did not look good. When I plugged it into Google Translate, this is what I read: "Hello! Since you are a foreign interview people, we consulted the relevant departments of the municipal government to accept any foreign interview to speak both official approval is required, so temporarily can not meet your requirements! Inconvenience, Please make alternative arrangements! Unfortunately!"

It was a nice note, I thought. But, of course, I went anyway.

CSPC was gated and guarded, but three men were taking a smoke break out in front. All wore the company uniform: a gray jacket with the CSPC logo and gray or navy blue pants. One offered me a smoke. They agreed to talk, but said anything official would have to go through a PR person for the company.

They confirmed that I had found the caffeine plant and said they also produced other associated chemicals. When I asked if they knew if it was the largest in the world, one man said yes, he knew it was the largest in the world. When I asked if it was modern and sophisticated on the inside, they said yes, it was.

I was at a loss. So I pulled out an energy shot that I had brought along. I handed it to one of the men and said it was made with Chinese caffeine and that the product was very popular in the United States. He asked if the caffeine had come from this plant. I said I did not think so. He shrugged, nonplussed, and handed it back to me.

My translator noticed that the men were a bit nervous as we spoke. They were looking over my shoulder at a young security officer in an olive green uniform, who had walked out to stand at the curb and watch them talk to me. We thanked them and walked off.

We poked around the neighborhood a bit more, attracting some stares and even a few handshakes, which my translator surmised might be because people were not used to seeing a Westerner in the neighborhood. And then we left.

⚡

Each caffeine plant likely synthesizes its caffeine in slightly different ways, but the basic steps are the same. BASF gave me a flow chart of its process. It starts by combining urea and chloroacetic acid to produce an intermediate compound called uracil. They use the uracil to produce theophylline, a close cousin to caffeine that occurs naturally in cacao and tea. Caffeine is, in essence, methylated theophylline, so in the last step, BASF methylates this synthetic theophylline by adding methyl chloride. Voilà—pure synthetic caffeine.

Whatever its origins, the chemical compound in its pure form is exactly the same. From a physiological standpoint, it does not matter a bit whether caffeine is synthesized in a factory or extracted from organic tea leaves by happy workers who are paid a living wage.

Any caffeine, synthetic or natural, might have impurities. Those impurities could be healthful or harmful, or they could simply be strange. And that leads us to a weird property of synthetic caffeine. It sometimes glows. We know this courtesy of U.S. patent 2,584,839, Decreasing Fluorescence of Synthetic Caffeine. Pfizer researcher Jay S. Buckley wrote this in his 1950 patent application: "Caffeine prepared synthetically often has a considerable bluish fluorescence which appears both in the solid compound and in solutions thereof. . . . The increased fluorescence is most undesirable, since it is often transmitted to other products in which caffeine is utilized, to their marked disadvantage." The process to rinse the glow from caffeine is fairly simple, using sodium nitrite, acetic acid, sodium carbonate, and chloroform.

Buckley was not the only scientist studying synthetic caffeine. In 1961, Coca-Cola and Monsanto researchers separately published papers describing tests to determine whether caffeine was synthetic or natural in origin. In essence, they used carbon dating—caffeine extracted from plant materials like tea shows a younger carbon signature than synthetic caffeine (since the synthetic version's chemical precursors are derived from fossil fuels, its carbon atoms have been kicking around for eons).

It is easy to understand why Coca-Cola would want a test for internal use, to verify their caffeine sources. But Monsanto had shifted to synthetic caffeine production, so why bother developing a test?

Chemist William Knowles, a Nobel Prize recipient who spent much of his career working for Monsanto, provided the answer in an oral history for the Chemical Heritage Foundation:

> Coke, which is the big customer, was afraid that somebody would get onto that—that we were making our caffeine in Coke from urea. Sounded too much like urine, you know what I mean? And, this would really kill them. So, they said, "We can only buy natural caffeine." Well, the Germans, they said, "Our supply is a natural caffeine." Well, I had been on a trip to Germany and I told our management I did not think that the Germans were doing that. I think they were mislabeling it. . . . Coke said, "But they're labeling it that. If you will label it natural caffeine, we'll buy it." And, Monsanto, and good credit too, they would not mislabel it. They would not do that. And, so, we said, "Well, how can we prove that the German is not natural?" Well, Woodward said, "Well, it's easy. We'll send it up to Libby and have him carbon date it." And, sure enough, it came out of the coal mine, dead.

Knowles's comment that "it came out of the coal mine" refers to the older carbon isotopes associated with synthetic caffeine.

These days, caffeine comes from all across the globe. One flavoring supplier for the soft drink industry sells thirteen varieties of caffeine powder from seven countries, including synthetic caffeine from China, kosher caffeine extracted from coffee beans in Italy, caffeine extracted from tea leaves in India, and guarana powder from Brazil. Increasingly, we get our synthetic caffeine fix from China. Just three Chinese factories exported seven million pounds of synthetic caffeine to the United States in 2011, nearly half of our total imports.

Most bottlers are cagey about their caffeine and reluctant to divulge their sources. They do this for two reasons: to keep their supply chains confidential and to downplay the association with chemicals perceived to be unnatural. Coca-Cola gave me this vague answer: "The caffeine that is used in our products comes from suppliers located in multiple geographies." Vivarin, which sells over-the-counter caffeine pills, said only, "It is the same type that is naturally occurring." Monster, at least, comes clean—it says its caffeine is synthetic.

Some bottlers are starting to tout the origins of their caffeine, as Maximus president Carlos de Aldecoa Bueno told me, but only if it is natural. Minute Maid, a Coca-Cola company, was doing so for a while. Minute Maid Enhanced juice drink carried this label: "Contains 37–43 mg of natural caffeine per bottle for an energy lift." (The label was also notable because Coca-Cola boasted of the energy lift, not just the flavor, provided by the same amount of caffeine in a Coke or Diet Coke.) Coca-Cola eventually discontinued this line of caffeinated juice drinks, but others have been waving the natural caffeine banner.

Ocean Spray has been advertising its CranErgy cranberry energy juice drink, boasting that it is "enhanced with natural caffeine from green tea extract." Frava ("fruit plus java"), another caffeinated fruit juice, launched in New York in early 2013, goes one step further, taking aim at synthetic caffeine on its Web site: "Most sodas and energy drinks use synthetic caffeine produced in a laboratory. Synthetic stimulants can be addictive and harmful. Frava cares about what you put in your body. That's why we use a natural source of caffeine from green coffee beans. Natural caffeine can increase brain functionality and alertness. It is used by our best athletes."

A Brazilian company run by entrepreneur Luis Goldner is hoping to cash in on the interest in natural caffeine. In 2011, Florida governor Rick Scott announced that America's Natural Caffeine will build a $25 million plant in Palm Beach to extract the drug from Brazilian gua-rana. Goldner even trademarked the phrase "ANC America's natural caffeine." But this well-hyped endeavor, which promised seventy-five jobs paying an average salary of sixty-two thousand dollars, may have buckled when faced with the market realities that favor producing caf-feine overseas. By early 2013, the company seemed to have gone AWOL.

Picking up where the Coca-Cola and Monsanto researchers left off fifty years earlier, a team of German researchers used carbon isotope analysis and liquid chromatography to determine the chemical signa-tures of various sources of caffeine and develop a finely tuned test to distinguish between natural and synthetic caffeine. Their research, published in 2011, showed that four out of thirty-eight products claiming to contain natural caffeine appeared to be adulterated with synthetic caffeine. These included two tea drinks and a maté drink. It is not surprising that some companies might mislabel the products—synthetic caffeine is cheaper, but "natural caffeine" sounds better to consumers. It was surprising, though, that they found an instant cof-fee that appeared to be boosted with synthetic caffeine.

If you want to ensure that your soft drink is made from natural caffeine, you can just buy it in Japan. The Ministry of Health, Labour, and Welfare's rather stringent regulations on food additives only al-low caffeine extract as defined this way: "A substance composed mainly of caffeine obtained from coffee beans or tea leaves."

⚡

After I left Shijiazhuang, I found that I was not alone in being turned away from CSPC. The caffeine plant also turned away inspectors for the European Directorate for the Quality of Medicines and HealthCare (EDQM). The agency withdrew the company's certification, losing CSPC a major caffeine market. By 2013, EDQM had withdrawn or suspended the certification of four out of five major caffeine suppliers in China.

Inspectors from the United States do not often visit the foreign plants like CSPC that supply so many of our pharmaceuticals. A 2007 General Accountability Office report estimated that the FDA would need thirteen years to inspect all such facilities (assuming no new ones came on line). By contrast, it inspected domestic pharmaceutical plants every two and a half years, on average. In 2008, the FDA got a wake-up call when tainted heparin (a blood thinner) produced in China was associated with eighty-one deaths in the United States. By 2011, the GAO said the FDA had increased its inspections, but it still faced major challenges. The GAO stated, "FDA faces limits on its ability to require foreign establishments to allow it to inspect their facilities. Furthermore, logistical issues preclude FDA from conducting unannounced inspections as it does for domestic establishments."

The congressional watchdog also noted that the FDA had incorrect information about foreign establishments in its databases and did not even know how many foreign companies were manufacturing drugs for the U.S. market. In its budget request for fiscal year 2014, the agency asked for a funding increase of $4.7 million to beef up its inspections of drug manufacturers in China.

The FDA did make the time to inspect one synthetic caffeine plant in Jilin province, in August 2009, and did not like what it saw. It took nine months for the agency to issue a warning letter to Jilin Shulan Synthetic Pharmaceutical Co. Even with its redactions, the FDA's May 2010 letter is good reading:

> Our investigator observed accumulated debris within wall
> and floor joints throughout your **REDACTED** USP

production facility. You used adhesive tape around hoses in the **REDACTED** and **REDACTED** rooms that became covered in production material. The **REDACTED** routinely spills onto the floor of the **REDACTED** rooms, causing the undersurfaces of your **REDACTED** to become rusty and caked with production materials. The investigator also observed **REDACTED** accumulation on the rusty stairs in the **REDACTED** room. When your personnel cleaned the **REDACTED** area in response to our investigator's comments regarding caked material on the underside of the **REDACTED** your personnel used mops soaked in dirty water.

And there was more:

During this inspection, the investigator observed individuals in the "**REDACTED** Clean Area" (including **REDACTED** areas) with open toe or open foot sandals, torn plastic booties, wearing no masks and wearing no gloves. We are concerned that you have not assessed the adequacy of these practices during drug manufacturing operations, particularly during the latter steps of **REDACTED** USP manufacturing.

The letter also highlights one unusual aspect of caffeine production and regulation. Caffeine is sometimes sold as a drug (using the acronym USP, for United States Pharmacopeia, or API, for Active Pharmaceutical Ingredient) and sometimes as a flavoring agent or food-grade chemical. It is the same product, often produced by the same plants, but the USP designation requires another layer of FDA scrutiny. Plants that produce only food-grade chemicals see less regulatory scrutiny. So Jilin Shulan, which used "mops soaked in dirty water," was at the top of the regulatory heap, producing prescription-grade caffeine.

In its letter, the FDA warned that, barring corrective action, "the articles could be subject to refusal of admission." Within a year, Jilin Shulan was on the FDA's Red List, which allows field personnel to detain drugs from firms that have not met "good manufacturing practices." While the redactions in the warning letter make it hard to determine which USP product was spilling onto the floor, the Red List details make it clear—it was caffeine. Like all its counterparts in China, the company's Web site shows a gleaming facility, with brightly lit white walls. But Jilin Shulan was producing caffeine in a filthy factory.

After the inspection, the plant shipped many tons of its product to an all-American company: Coca-Cola. After the FDA issued its warning, but before the company landed on the Red List, Coca-Cola bought more than one hundred thousand pounds of caffeine from Jilin Shulan— enough to make 1.3 billion cans of Coke. (Like most of the corporation's caffeine, it was routed through its wholly owned subsidiary Caribbean Refrescos, a plant in Puerto Rico that produces soft drink concentrates.)

When I asked Coca-Cola why it was still buying caffeine from the plant fifteen months after the FDA inspection showed unsanitary conditions, it responded with this statement: "All our ingredients, products and packaging are safe. This is the most important commitment we make. Upon learning of the issuance of a warning letter resulting from a previous FDA inspection of the Jilin facility, we immediately cancelled all pending purchases of caffeine from that supplier."

Dr Pepper was another Jilin Shulan customer. When Cadbury Schweppes owned Dr Pepper, it even highlighted the plant in a 2004 report on social responsibility.

"Jilin Shulan Pharmaceutical Company in China is a long term contract supplier of caffeine, a flavour concentrate ingredient used widely in beverages including our own Dr Pepper beverage," the report stated. "Shulan began to produce and export caffeine in 1987 after Pfizer withdrew from the market. . . . Dr Pepper began to purchase caffeine from this factory in 2001 after the plant passed a facility audit in November 2000."

In other words, Jilin Shulan, where the FDA found filthy conditions in 2009, was not just a rogue, fringe pharmaceutical plant. It was a plant that had been touted by one of the world's largest beverage corporations, just five years earlier, as the exemplar of a good, long-term source of caffeine. Either Dr Pepper was hyping a marginal plant in 2004, or the plant went downhill quickly over the next five years.

And that is the nub of what I learned in Shijiazhuang: The industry is opaque, and the little information that is publicly available is not reassuring. But until they are inspected, it is impossible to document any problems at the caffeine plants. And because inspections are quite rare, American consumers have little assurance that the caffeine in their sodas comes from clean pharmaceutical plants.

Unlike heparin, which is used intravenously, it would take a lot of impurities to make caffeine sufficiently contaminated to harm people, but these days, when so many people know not only the variety of tomatoes they prefer but also the name of the farm or maybe even the farmer who produced them, we remain uninformed about the origins of the caffeine in America's favorite caffeinated beverages. With the exception of those who work in the caffeine industry, all of my sources—regulators, researchers, and chemists—were under the same misperception as the rest of us. They believed that most caffeine is derived from decaffeination.

Not only are most of us naive about how caffeine is produced; we know little about how it is blended into consumer products. That is why I went to New Jersey.

CHAPTER 9

From Stacker to Sunkist

High in the hills of northwestern New Jersey, along the Lackawanna ridge, is a tranquil rural region, where dairy farms are nestled alongside rocky, wooded hills, and swans swim in small ponds on spring mornings. One especially scenic farm, Mooney's Dairy, has a red barn, green John Deere tractors, and a sign touting its registered Holsteins. Just across the road, at the site of a former cheese factory, is NVE Pharmaceuticals. This is the source of two of the nation's best-selling energy shots. The company claims $50 million in sales annually, 90 percent of which comes from caffeinated products.

When I arrived at the office on the second floor of the factory, the receptionist seemed to be having trouble with a customer on the phone.

"Just take the bottle with you," she said. "The package is the proof; it's all listed on the ingredients." On the wall was a six-foot poster for caffeine pills, reading, "Stacker 2, World's Strongest Fat Burner." Earlier ad campaigns had featured cast members of another well-known New Jersey export: *The Sopranos*.

When the receptionist hung up, I told her I was there to see Walter Orcutt. She called him, then asked me to sit on a couch while I waited and said, "Do you want a coffee or something, water?" I'd half-expected her to offer me a caffeine pill, or at least an energy shot.

Orcutt came out to meet me. NVE's executive vice president, he is a friendly, energetic, and effusive man in his fifties. He said it was a good day to tour the plant, because he was also showing around a visitor from South America, who was having an energy drink bottled that day, and a blending guru who worked as a flavor consultant in the Midwest.

First, he showed us to a room at the front of the plant, where the raw materials start the conversion to energy products and other caffeine delivery mechanisms. A large blending machine topped by a funnel-shaped hopper stands in the center of the room. The caffeine goes into the hopper, along with any other dry flavors and vitamins, to be sifted and blended. The bulk product, a "slippery powder," then goes into big blue barrels.

From there, we walked through a door into a room where three men were tending a pill press. A Hispanic temporary worker was using a bucket to dip the caffeine/vitamin powder from a fifty-five-gallon blue barrel and pour it into the top of a pill press. Orcutt told us the plant employs seventy people, with another fifty to a hundred temps daily.

The press was rhythmically thumping out a stream of capsules—half-yellow, half-blue—each packing two hundred milligrams of caffeine and sold as dietary and energy supplements.

Admiring the pill operation, the energy drink maker asked Orcutt, "Do you need any FDA approval for this?"

"You don't need approval first, no."

"Not like a drug."

"No, not like that," said Orcutt.

He took us over to an area where the pills were lined up on a machine and pressed into a blister pack. There was a steady *whoomp, tock, whoomp, tock* as the blister packer sealed them, four to a pack. The air smelled faintly of hot plastic. After being sealed, each package is stamped with an American flag and the words "Made in USA." These caffeine pills are sold in convenience stores. "We kind of own that market," Orcutt said.

An earlier pill formulation nearly sunk the company. Diet pills combining caffeine and ephedra caused heart problems and even fatalities. The drug combination became national news when Baltimore Orioles pitcher Steve Bechler collapsed and died at spring training in February 2003 and an autopsy cited ephedra as a factor (he had taken supplements made by one of NVE's competitors). NVE was hit with more than 110 product liability lawsuits over its caffeine-ephedra supplements.

The ephedra problems prompted congressional hearings in 2003, where FDA commissioner Mark McClellan talked about the perils. "In September 2002, FDA became aware of the tragic death of Sean Riggins, the sixteen-year-old high school football player who had taken the product Yellow Jackets," said McClellan. "The product was manufactured by NVE Pharmaceuticals in New Jersey. Yellow Jacket capsules and Black Beauty capsules, another NVE product at the time, were both 'street' terms for controlled substances, and are sold as herbal street drug alternatives. These products are labeled to contain ephedra extract and other herbal ingredients, including kola nut extract, a source of caffeine."

When the FDA had tried to inspect NVE in October 2002, the company turned the inspectors away. They returned with U.S. Marshals, and in January 2003 they watched NVE voluntarily destroy street-drug alternative products worth nearly $5 million. But McClellan said the company did little to alter its practices and continued to pump out pills that looked like speed. "After NVE stopped marketing Yellow Jackets and Black Beauties, they began marketing Yellow Swarm and Midnight Stallion as replacement products," he said. "These products appear to be almost identical in formulation and appearance, but they no longer bear street-drug names or claims—yet safety issues associated with these types of products remain."

As we passed the pill-packing line, Orcutt told me the company went into Chapter 11 for two years after the ephedra controversy, then settled in a class action for $20 million. But he insisted that the product had merit as a diet pill.

"That was killer; the ephedra was a really good product," Orcutt told me. But he said people were just taking too much. "People were blowing their hearts out." One vestige of the era is the name "stacker" on so many NVE products. It refers to the ephedrine, caffeine, and aspirin combination, a.k.a. an ECA stack, which was once a popular weight-loss formula. The company still sells Yellow Swarm pills, but now they are ephedra-free; caffeine alone gives them their kick.

⚡

The real action was farther back in the building, in a room with three lines for bottling energy shots. With a rhythmic *clink, whoosh, plonk*, energy shots—white plastic bottles shrink-wrapped in purple—went snaking in long lines through the cavernous room.

Orcutt said NVE's 6 Hour Power is the second-best-selling energy shot in the United States, and its Stacker 2 Xtra brand is the top-selling energy shot at dollar stores. 5-hour Energy pioneered the energy shot concept, and NVE, looking to diversify from caffeine pills, followed close behind. NVE's energy shots first gained traction in Walgreens; by 2012 it had more than seven different products on the shelves in Walmart.

The empty vials landed in a spinning steel tub that oriented them. After a machine stamped a batch code and best-by date on the bottom, the vials marched upright, single file, to a station where tubes squirted them full of caffeinated liquid. Because the liquid is viscous, NVE had to specially modify the filler tubes from materials used in the cosmetics industry. Once the bottles were filled, a machine dropped on the plastic sleeve with the label. With a whoosh, the shots were wrapped and the plastic perforated for easy opening. At the end of the line, twelve vials were packed to a cardboard tray that doubles as a display stand.

Orcutt pulled a vial off the line to show us. "This is the dollar store product. So we don't have to package it as well, because they don't market them well," he said. "We do more than a hundred thousand bottles per line, per eight-hour shift."

That's more than six million shots a month, each two-ounce vial incorporating about 150 to 175 milligrams of caffeine (two SCADs). Put another way, these shots alone account for forty 55-pound boxes of China white every month.

Orcutt uses the stuff himself. "I'll pound coffee all day long," he told me, "but at the end of the day, I'll slam a shot." Still, he said he was surprised at the demand for the energy shots made by NVE and its competitors. "It's crazy, it makes no sense—three dollars for a shot. But that's the way it is."

NVE may be the number two energy shot in the country, but it is a distant second to the top dog in energy shots. 5-hour Energy was selling $1 billion worth of caffeinated syrup annually by 2012. Both companies have elbowed out the competition in the market for small vials of liquid caffeine. Monster developed its own energy shot, called Hitman, and Rockstar had its own label. Both flopped. The big boys also got into the game. Coke developed NOS energy shots and Pepsi developed Amp energy shots. They crashed, too. But the billions to be made with energy drinks and shots did effectively bring Coke and Pepsi out of the caffeine closet—Coca-Cola bottles Full Throttle and NOS energy drinks and Pepsi bottles Amp energy drinks. The companies are coming full circle, acknowledging caffeine's pharmacological appeal and going back to their roots selling America's first energy drinks.

Orcutt took us outside and across a parking lot to see the bottling line, which occupies another large building. At the front of the building is a small flavor-blending lab: a table with beakers on a drying rack, shot glasses and little Dixie cups, and a bottle of ShopRite sodium-free seltzer.

Just beyond the tasting lab is a vast room where thousands of cans of energy drinks chugged along a line that meandered here and there like a continuous model train. Walking through the plant was a bit like being at a music festival, hearing new sounds as you wander from stage to stage. Over here it was the *whomp-chuck* of the lids being tamped on, here the *tick, tick, tick* of the cans stutter-stepping through the warehouse. Every once in a while, these were punctuated with a big spraying sound, as the mixing tank relieved pressure. The air was lightly fogged with a sweet, caffeinated mist.

Stacked against a wall on one side of the room were the ingredients: boxes of dry mix and five- and fifty-gallon barrels of wet mix. When blending an energy drink or a cola, each variety has its own recipe: ten bags of this dry mix, say, and two buckets of that wet mix. It all goes into a large vat to be blended with water and then carbonated. The caffeine is typically part of the dry mix.

NVE produces energy drinks on contract to private labels. So if you want a product called Green Flash to sell in the Virgin Islands, or Colombian Power for export to Colombia, NVE will conceive, concoct, and can it for you. Orcutt said NVE has exported energy drinks all over the world, to Lebanon, Australia, Syria, and Russia (where it is tough to get paid). Stacked high overhead on one end of the warehouse were cases and cases of energy drinks made for different labels. There were Rush and Impulse energy drinks, and Playboy and Penthouse, and Sum Poosie, packaged for strip clubs and illustrated with busty women in bikinis ("It's perfect, want sum, need sum, get sum."). Judging from what was there in the warehouse, it seemed as though every commercial sector wanted a piece of the energy drink action.

⚡

You might remember the energy drink with a name that incited the FDA's ire: Cocaine. NVE cans that, too. To illustrate how strange federal regulations can be, Orcutt picked up a can of Cocaine and read the warning label that regulators had signed off on: "WARNING: This message is for the people who are too stupid to recognize the obvious. This product does not contain cocaine (duh). This product is not intended to be an alternative to an illicit street drug, and anyone who thinks otherwise is an idiot."

As we toured the bottling plant, Orcutt was running a three-thousand-case shift of energy drinks for export to South America. Walking past a part of the line where the cans, already filled, were awaiting their lids, he said, "Here, try this." He snagged a can as it filed past and handed it to me. It tasted great—cold, sweet, and fizzy, with the faint, bitter tang of caffeine.

Pure caffeine is the essence of bitter. Scientists studying taste often use caffeine to understand reactions to bitter flavors. Flavoring houses even sell caffeine-masking agents to hide the flavor, but it is not always easy. To diminish its taste in a dissolvable film, Roger Stier, at the New Jersey flavoring house Noville Inc., uses a three-step process: "We selected the Cremophor RH 40 [a variety of hydrogenated castor oil made by BASF] to coat the taste receptors and added citric acid to compete within the channel receptors with the bitter stimuli. Sucralose was selected as the sweetener. . . . When the three-part masking system was added to the finished films, the bitterness of the caffeine was significantly reduced."

After the other visitors had left, I asked Orcutt to show me the caffeine. We walked to a large, dark storeroom at the side of the building, where boxes and barrels of flavoring agents were stored. From a distance, he gestured toward a tall stack of boxes back by the loading dock.

We walked down there, and sure enough, dozens of fifty-five-pound boxes of caffeine, eighteen to a pallet, were stacked overhead. It was the good stuff, packed in a container in China, shipped to the Port of New York and New Jersey, then trucked over to NVE. Pure synthetic caffeine. China white.

Seeing the caffeine-packaging process in NVE's bottling plant helped me understand a story that I'd been interested in since I visited Texas.

On September 28, 2010, Robert Callan realized he had a problem. Callan was the senior vice president of Dr Pepper Snapple Group, and customers had been calling his office at company headquarters in Plano, Texas, complaining about a medicinal flavor in their Sunkist sodas. One caller said it tasted like baby aspirin and caused stomach pains. Others had it worse, throwing up and even going to the hospital overnight.

The next day, Callan notified the Food and Drug Administration that he was recalling 4,382 cases of Sunkist bottled in twelve-ounce plastic bottles. He dispatched employees to gather more than 105,000 bottles from stores in Nebraska, Oklahoma, and Texas. Then Callan fired the three employees who had bungled the blend, retrained several others, corresponded with the FDA, and moved on.

Sunkist is an orange soda. It started out as a partnership between the Sunkist citrus-growers cooperative and General Cinema. It was test-marketed in 1978 and formally launched in 1979. An aggressive advertising campaign, led by New York's Foote, Cone & Belding, included TV spots showing tanned, athletic youths frolicking on skimboards, surfboards, and catamarans to the tune of the Beach Boys' "Good Vibrations." Sunkist broke into the nation's top ten soft drinks within a year and was the leading orange soda for more than a decade. It has since gone through several hands, but now Sunkist is bottled by Dr Pepper Snapple Group, the third-largest soft drink bottler in the United States, behind Coke and Pepsi.

Third place is plenty big in the soft drink business. Dr Pepper Snapple Group's net sales in the United States exceeded $5 billion in 2012. It sells 1.6 billion cases of beverages annually—enough for every man, woman, and child in the United States to drink 180 twelve-ounce bottles. Sunkist is its best-selling orange soda. It might surprise you to know that it has an ingredient common to all of the top five soft drinks in the United States and eight of the top ten: caffeine.

Many people think of orange soda as a drink for kids. And most do not think of Sunkist as a caffeinated drink. But it contains forty-one milligrams of caffeine per twelve-ounce bottle—more than a Coke but less than a Mountain Dew. A twenty-ounce bottle packs a SCAD.

The consumer complaints Callan was fielding were caused by a batch of Sunkist bottled on September 4, 2010. The soda was blended with caffeine levels that were not just high, but off the charts.

Each twelve-ounce bottle was dosed with 238 milligrams, as much as three Red Bulls or sixteen ounces of strong coffee—three SCADs. That is a stout dose for an adult habituated to caffeine. It is a whopping dose for a twelve-year-old, not to mention a toddler with a sippy cup. Instead of good vibrations, the sodas were packing bad jitters.

Callan downplayed the concerns in his correspondence with the FDA. In a September 29 letter, he wrote: "There have been 11 consumer inquiries about the Product which focused upon its medicinal flavor. The caffeine level was not consumer perceptible, but was discovered after we investigated the flavor inquiries."

Here is part of the log of one consumer's complaint, phoned in on September 28 and later relayed to the FDA: "I bought an 8pk of Sunkist Orange and we all got sick. My son is in the hospital. Me, my son and my nephew drank some. My 12 yr old son drank a bottle. I gave some to my 18 month old nephew and mixed with water in his sippy cup. Fifteen minutes after my son drank the bottle he started feeling dizzy, had a fever of 100 and stated [sic] throwing up. I took my son to the hospital last night. He is still at the hospital and he is doing better."

The consumer signed off, saying her lawyer would be sending a letter. The account raises some questions about the consumer's judgment. But it also suggests Callan's assertion that the caffeine was not consumer perceptible was a bit of a stretch.

At least two other customers complained of getting sick. Comments about the flavor included: "kind of tasted like medicine"; tasted like baby aspirin; and "wasn't like sour but it tasted bad." To assuage one concerned customer, the company "apologized and sent 1-12 pack coupon. . . . Settled with coupon."

The FDA's Shirley Spitler sent Callan a few questions via e-mail. Among them: "Has your firm determined what the root cause of the mis-labeling was?"

Callan replied, "A **REDACTED** gallon batching kit was misapplied in a **REDACTED** gallon batching kit on 9/4." Reading between the lines, the cause looks pretty simple—a bottling plant employee mixed in six times as much caffeine as he should have.

This snafu was clearly enough to cause acute discomfort for some consumers, but not enough caffeine to cause a fatal overdose. But it is hard to know what the health consequences were, because the FDA did not do any follow-up. Further, the recall was not announced in public media (in fact, it has never before been reported), so it is likely that some consumers noticed the effects but did not know to attribute them to the high-caffeine Sunkist.

Some energy drink aficionados might like to get their hands on a bottle of the super-Sunkist, but they are out of luck. Dr Pepper Snapple destroyed 3,254 cases of the Sunkist—74 percent of the bungled batch—on October 13 and 14, 2010. But the incident provided a rare glimpse through the keyhole at the blending practices of one of the nation's top soft-drink bottlers, all of whom are private, if not secretive, about their industrial practices.

Another glimpse came just eight months later, in an incident at another Dr Pepper Snapple Group bottling plant. That time, the bottler recalled a diet cola bottled for Walgreens.

Mislabeled "caffeine free" instead of "calorie free," twelve thousand cases of the cola hit shelves nationwide, with about seventy-five milligrams of caffeine in each twenty-ounce bottle (the specified amount of caffeine for the standard version of the cola). That is one SCAD on the nose, a bit less than an eight-ounce Red Bull, and sufficient to get the attention of anyone who is sensitive to caffeine's effects. After a customer complained to Walgreen's, the labeling mixup prompted another voluntary recall.

Notably, the FDA ranked the latter recall as a more serious problem. The Walgreens recall was a Class II recall: "a situation in which use of or exposure to a violative product may cause temporary or medically reversible adverse health consequences or where the probability of serious adverse health consequences is remote."

The supercharged Sunkist only warranted a Class III recall: "a situation in which use of or exposure to a violative product is not likely to cause adverse health consequences." (It is hard to understand the rationale for ranking the Sunkist incident lower, except that people who are particularly caffeine sensitive and want to avoid it altogether might have been at risk from the Walgreens soda; the Sunkist, by contrast, is a matter of degrees since the consumers had chosen to buy a caffeinated soda.)

When I asked to tour the Dr Pepper Snapple plant in Irving, Texas, to see how the company had changed its process to prevent another such fiasco, Chris Barnes, the manager of corporate affairs, replied in an e-mail: "There was nothing that needed to be changed with respect to process and procedure. We produce many millions of cases of beverages with caffeine each year out of that one facility in Irving with no issue. The issue leading to the voluntary recall of that single run of Sunkist was an error in the batching process. We've reinforced existing procedures with our staff and there have been no similar issues since."

Actually, the company did change its process and procedure, according to a Corrective Action Memo it sent to the FDA in January 2011. In addition to terminating three employees, including one who not only failed to taste the samples but falsified documentation to state otherwise, the company stepped up its batcher training and agreed to reduce employee rotation in the ingredient room and improve its storage of ingredients. Under "caffeine testing," it agreed to "add Sunkist testing for caffeine to prove consistency of production, particularly during the batch training process."

Because caffeine recalls are rare and Dr Pepper Snapple had had two in just six months, I also asked Barnes about the Walgreens recall. He replied: "The other issue you've brought up with the Walgreens cola, which we produce on a contract basis, was not related to the product itself, but rather the labels provided by the label supplier. As with the Sunkist issue, we handled this to the satisfaction of the FDA."

It's true. The FDA signed off on the voluntary recalls. While not disinterested, it did not appear preoccupied by the super-caffeination or the mislabeling. When FDA regulators did become interested in caffeine, it was not sodas that caught their attention, but newly developed caffeine delivery mechanisms. But that was still a couple of years away.

PART III

CAFFEINATED BODY, CAFFEINATED BRAIN

CHAPTER 10

The Athletes' Favorite Drug

At four thirty on a warm October morning, I stopped by Kona Brothers Coffee, in Kona, Hawaii. As I paid for my sixteen-ounce cup of locally grown, medium-roast coffee, the barista said, "We'll be here to caffeinate you all day." It was the café's busiest day of the year, and he'd already pulled an all-nighter.

By five, I was sitting on the nearby seawall. Waves were lapping six feet below, and lights showed the route of shorefront Ali'i Drive, off to my left, wrapping around the bay to a geometric hotel profiled on a point. Behind the hotel, scattered house lights outlined the shape of the mountain that rises directly from the sea, fading in the distance to the stars above, where Orion stood, dead vertical overhead, above a low-hanging fingernail moon.

All around me, thousands of spectators jostled for the best seats on the seawall. Looking down the wall from where I sat, I could see a long line of legs draped over the edge, and between nearly every pair of knees, a hand cradled a cup of coffee. I sat there in the warm ocean breeze, sipping my Kona, which was fantastic, whether or not it tasted like a middling Central American coffee, as Michael Norton had so profitably understood.

Off to my right, two hundred yards across the harbor, a brightly lit pier was bustling. Hundreds of people scurried to and fro, clad in Lycra and neoprene. By six a.m., day was breaking, announcers' voices began booming over the PA systems, and the first competitors waded tentatively into the water to start warming up.

It was the start of an annual ritual. Every year, many of the planet's fittest athletes converge in Kona for the Ironman World Championship. It is a brutal triathlon: a 2.4-mile swim in the Pacific swells, followed by a 112-mile bike ride on a road flanked by lava fields, topped off by a marathon. You have to earn the privilege to race at Kona, and even that isn't easy. The nineteen hundred athletes competing in 2012 had taken the top few spots at qualifying triathlons all across the globe.

First in the water were the crème de la crème of these elite athletes, the professionals. By 6:20, the pro men's field was warming up, crowding the starting line between a pair of markers as volunteers on paddleboards and in kayaks herded them back. Finally, a cannon shot signaled the race's start, the crowd roared, and the racers churned the water into a froth.

Ten minutes later, it was the pro women's turn. It was a small field—just thirty-one pro women had qualified for the race. Sarah Piampiano was among them. Though just a first-year pro, Piampiano had already won an Ironman race in New Orleans and was the second American woman at the 2012 Ironman U.S. Championship in Manhattan.

With another cannon shot, the women were off. Soon they were out of the harbor, swimming past a float serving free Kona coffee and heading for the distant turnaround. In their wakes, the real chaos began, as eighteen hundred amateur triathletes, the "age-groupers," jostled for the start. Most were jacked up on caffeine, the world's most popular performance-enhancing drug.

⚡

The day before the Kona race, Piampiano was relaxing in a friend's house, high above the endorphinated madness down in town, drinking a calorie-rich smoothie and telling me about her caffeine strategy. "While I'm racing, caffeine is actually a pretty important part of my day," she said. "Particularly in the Ironman, where it's such a long race, and you are competing over nine to ten hours."

Piampiano is not a caffeine addict. She has maybe two cups of coffee in a year, because she is sensitive to its effects. It makes her jittery. But on race day, she uses it thoughtfully and systematically to optimize her performance. She uses energy gels made by Clif Bar, one of her sponsors, to integrate calories and caffeine into her race-day nutrition plan. Before the race, she usually takes a gel with fifty milligrams of caffeine. Then on the biking leg, she takes fifty milligrams per hour. And that increases later in the race.

Piampiano spread out a variety of her energy products on a coffee table. "Here I've got some Clif Shot Bloks, which are actually kind of like gummy bears almost. They are kind of jelly in consistency." She uses the blocks during the biking leg, when it is easier to chew. She also had several energy gels—which have the consistency of thick honey and come in foil pouches—to use during the run. Throughout the day, she tries to take about three hundred calories per hour and augments that with increasing doses of caffeine.

"As you get further into the marathon, your energy supplies are depleted and you just really start suffering, and that's why I start increasing the amount of caffeine I take. At the end of the marathon, you need that energy kick," she said. And Piampiano said caffeine is an essential tool for an elite triathlete. "It's critical, particularly if you want to perform and have any success at the top level."

By seven thirty, the professional racers were trickling back in to the harbor, first the men, then the women. Piampiano completed the swim in just over an hour, in a small group including Natascha Badmann, a six-time Kona champion. They sprinted up a ramp past cheering throngs, stripped off their wetsuits, strapped on their cycling shoes and aerodynamic, teardrop-shaped helmets, and mounted their carbon fiber bikes for the 112-mile ride.

A few minutes later, I watched Piampiano pump up a hill in town. She wore a red and black Lycra outfit emblazoned with her sponsors' logos. On her biceps, she wore rub-on Clif tattoos. Her bike was a Cervélo P5, a wind-shearing, six-thousand-dollar wonder. She carried water bottles on her down tube and handlebars and another behind her seat. And tucked into the pockets of her jersey were the energy blocks—the caffeinated gummy bears—she would so methodically chew for the next five hours.

She was out of the saddle, looking determined, cranking up the hill, planning to stick with Badmann. But soon the relentless winds and heat of the lava fields sapped her energy. Badmann—sponsored by caffeine drink pioneer Red Bull—was on fire (she would post the fastest bike time of the day). Feeling lousy, Piampiano fell off Badmann's pace. In an effort to restore her flagging energy, she started drinking Coke at every aid station, in addition to her precisely calibrated nutrient and caffeine plan.

Though she was suffering, she turned in what most cyclists would consider a blistering time for the leg, averaging more than 20 miles per hour for 112 miles. Then she laced up her running shoes for the real fun—26.2 miles through the humid Hawaiian heat.

Using her caffeinated energy gels, Piampiano was in good company. Most of the super-fit endurance athletes at Kona used caffeine, but there were as many different strategies, it seemed, as there were racers.

A forty-five-year-old amateur from Ontario told me she usually has just one cup of coffee in the morning. But on race day she also takes two caffeinated gels during the bike ride and two caffeine pills just before the run.

Warming up by the seawall the day before the race, Sam Gydé, of Belgium, told me he takes a less systematic approach to caffeine. "I have a very busy life and a very busy work, and I train a lot, so I just drink lots of coffee. So I am naturally very caffeinated. During training and racing I use gels, which contain caffeine, and it's not with any purpose," he said with a shrug, "but I'm more or less like a heavy caffeine user." (I watched Gydé cross the finish line in nine hours and six minutes, looking fresh as a daisy and winning the thirty-five to thirty-nine age group for the second year running.)

But not everyone is on board. Daniel Fontana is a professional racer. An Argentine by birth, he represents Italy, where he has lived for ten years. "For me, it's not very good to take caffeine during the races," Fontana said. "I have stomach problems. Mostly in a very hot race, it can irritate my stomach. So I will use my own gels, my own drinking system, and I will try to avoid caffeine during the race."

Peter Vervoort, an MD from Belgium, has studied caffeine in athletes in Antwerp. He said for many athletes in his studies, doses of 200 to 350 milligrams were not helpful, especially in hot weather. He also competed in the Ironman and told me, "I'm not using caffeine. I do use Coca-Cola in the last twenty kilometers. But that's caffeine in very small doses." He said it's actually getting hard to avoid caffeine on the race course. "There are more and more gel companies which only make gels with caffeine. So it is difficult."

Vervoort is an outlier. Most researchers have come to a different conclusion about caffeine's ergogenic effects. And the research started a century ago.

As long ago as 1909, endurance athletes were singing the praises of Coca-Cola. (Remember, in this era Coke had the same caffeine concentration as a modern Red Bull.) In a display ad that year, the track cyclist Bobby Walthour had this to say: "When I first went into a six-day race I took a jug of Coca-Cola to New York with me and drank it all the time I was there. I won the championship and came out of that great contest ten pounds heavier than when I went in. After that experience I have never been without Coca-Cola, because it keeps me fresh, but does not stimulate and then leave me all broken up." Gaining ten pounds over a six-day race sounds improbable, but it must have been, in those days, a selling point.

In 1912, several researchers from the University of Kansas Physiological Laboratory used Coca-Cola to study caffeine's effect on work capacity in two subjects, an athlete and a nonathlete.

The study was more of an oddity than a lasting contribution to caffeine science, but it's notable for several reasons: It was among the first to show that caffeine can increase work capacity in trained athletes; both subjects abstained from caffeine for several weeks before the experiment in order to eliminate the confounding nature of caffeine addiction; and it ended badly.

For most of the research, they used "7 ounces of coca-cola, containing a total of 1.42 grains of caffeine, being the average amount in a strong cup of coffee." That amount is roughly equal to ninety-two milligrams, which is a bit more than a SCAD. The scientists observed the number of repetitions the subjects could complete using weights with and without breakfast, and with and without caffeine.

In sum, the researchers found, "the conclusion of previous workers—that an optimum dose of caffeine increases the capacity for muscular work and inhibits the sense of fatigue and that a larger dose decreases the power for muscular contraction—was confirmed."

Among the many limitations of the study were the small number of subjects and their unique traits. Subject A was an untrained athlete and regular coffee drinker, five feet tall and 140 pounds. The second subject was a bear of a man, a physical education instructor standing five foot eight, weighing 196 pounds.

The researchers had hoped to do more research on the aftereffects of caffeine use, but that did not work out so well. "It was not possible to state how long the after effect would endure," they wrote, "because the experiments were suddenly interrupted by the paralysis of the rectus muscle of the left eye in the athlete and the nervous condition of the non-athlete."

It's worth taking a moment here to visualize a punching bag drill Subject B, the athlete, had perfected: "Before he began the experiments he had trained himself so that he was able to hit the punching bag with his head, feet and hands alternately on its rebound. It required speed, accuracy and control of muscles, and concentration of thought. But his power of concentration, accuracy and precision in his muscles had been greatly impaired so that he was unable to repeat the athletic demonstration with any credit during the time he was taking the strong doses of caffeine."

Given the subjects' unpleasant symptoms, the scientists abruptly abandoned their study. "The indications were that there were after effects which interfered with efficiency of physical and mental activities," they wrote.

The science seems antiquated now, because it is. But this novel set of experiments showing that caffeine reduced fatigue and increased power hinted at the research yet to come.

⚡

While in Kona, I tracked down Matthew Ganio, an exercise physiologist at the University of Arkansas Department of Health, Human Performance, and Recreation, and Evan Johnson, a University of Connecticut doctoral candidate. They have collaborated on caffeine research and were in Hawaii to study the effects of the triathlon on athletes' physiology.

Fair-haired and youthful, Ganio is soft-spoken, but he is unequivocal about caffeine's benefits for athletes. In 2009, Ganio and his colleagues published a systematic review of twenty-one studies on caffeine in timed performance. Most of the researchers looked at subjects cycling, but some also studied running, rowing, and cross-country skiing, and most of the tests were in the fifteen-minute to two-hour range. Looking across all the results, Ganio found consistent improvements in performance.

The improvements can be substantial, he told me, often as much as 3 percent. "There is always going to be some variability—some people won't see as much of an effect as others; some people will see a large effect. Some people may not like it as much, or it may impair their performance a little bit. But on average, it does improve performance," he said. Best of all, it is legal for nearly all sporting events.

To put that into context, a 3 percent improvement would mean an eighteen-minute boost in a ten-hour race. Eighteen minutes was all that separated the top eight finishers in both the men's and women's pro races at Kona.

For recreational athletes, too, the effects can be dramatic. A runner who is able to complete a 10K race in forty minutes without caffeine could shave off seventy-two seconds with caffeine. And caffeine could allow a cyclist competing in a one-hour time trial to drop a minute and a half.

"Caffeine is a very unique drug in that it has effects on almost every different part of the body," Ganio said. "The general consensus right now is that a lot of it is going on in the brain, or the central nervous system." Through antagonizing the neurotransmitter adenosine, which tells the brain when we are tired, it alleviates fatigue.

Ganio said it is important to take the right dose, which shakes out to about three to six milligrams per kilogram of body mass. That is a lot of caffeine. An eighty-kilo (176-pound) athlete taking six milligrams per kilogram would need 480 milligrams of caffeine. "That's four strong cups of coffee," said Ganio. "If you can tolerate it, it seems to be the upper end of what you can have to improve performance."

Since "cups of coffee" is a notoriously imprecise measure of caffeine, it may help to think of it this way: 480 milligrams would be six 8-ounce Red Bulls, two and a half NoDoz tablets, or two Extra Strength 5-hour Energy shots. It is more than six SCADs.

A more moderate dose for a smaller athlete, say, a sixty-five-kilo (143-pound) athlete taking three milligrams per kilo, is still an impressive amount of caffeine: two and a half SCADs, equal to one No-Doz tablet, one 5-hour Energy shot, or two and a half Red Bulls. Even this amount of caffeine is difficult to obtain using caffeinated sodas like Coca-Cola. A sixty-five-kilo athlete would need to chug nearly six cans of Coke at once to get a caffeine dose of three milligrams per kilogram.

But smaller doses of caffeine can sometimes prove quite effective.

In a study of competitive athletes cycling for two hours, low doses of caffeine late in the activity (1.5 milligrams per kilogram, consumed in Coca-Cola) proved effective in enhancing performance.

According to Ganio, most endurance athletes use caffeine. (That is partly because most people use caffeine daily, whether or not they are athletes.) But he said many athletes still have some misperceptions about caffeine. One of those is that it will dehydrate you.

One hydration study followed fifty-nine healthy male volunteers for eleven days, using varying levels of caffeine. The researchers found no evidence of dehydration. "These findings question the widely accepted notion that caffeine consumption acts chronically as a diuretic," the scientists concluded.

While this finding will seem counterintuitive to many coffee drinkers, especially commuters who have suffered through bladder-bursting traffic jams, Ganio said the science bears it out. Twelve ounces of coffee or twelve ounces of water will have about the same effect.

Ganio said people are also confused about whether they should abstain from caffeine in the days leading up to an athletic event, in order to maximize its effects. But he said there is not enough data about this. "As far as performance, it seems pretty clear that regardless of how much you are habituated to it, you can still see an effect." Still, he does recommend that athletes abstain from caffeine leading up to an event. Abstaining from caffeine for a week or so allows your brain to reset its adenosine receptors, reducing your tolerance and giving caffeine a greater effect at lower doses. Conversely, he said, it would be a bad idea for habituated users to think they should double up on caffeine to compensate for their daily use. This could put them above the optimal dose and into a range that could cause jitters or stomach trouble.

Athletes are all over the map on this issue. Very few athletes (like few adults in general) typically abstain from caffeine like Piampiano does. Kent Bostick, a cyclist who competed in the Olympics and has won United States championships, told me that caffeine gave him an edge. But he thinks it is because he otherwise abstained from caffeine and had no tolerance to it. "I would take a half of a Vivarin and a big tall cup of coffee. It gave me a pretty good kick for race day," he said. And he said the difference was notable to his peers, who used to ask him, "How come you go so much faster on race day?"

Still, it may not be essential to suffer through withdrawal to give yourself a boost on race day. A group of Australian researchers tested twelve male cyclists who were regular caffeine users. All received pills for the four days leading up to the trials. Some pills were placebos; others were caffeinated. The subjects then completed a one-hour cycling test. Caffeine improved performance just as much in the cyclists who'd been abstaining from caffeine as in those who had been taking it steadily. "No significant difference was detected between the two acute caffeine trials (placebo-caffeine vs. caffeine-caffeine)," the researchers wrote. "A 3 mg/kg dose of caffeine significantly improves exercise performance irrespective of whether a 4-day withdrawal period is imposed on habitual caffeine users."

Evan Johnson, Ganio's research colleague, who is dark-haired, fit, and energetic, said one limitation on caffeine research in athletes is that most studies have looked at shorter endurance events, typically an hour in length, and none have focused on caffeine's effects in Ironman-length races. As a former competitor, he knows something about the grueling events and said it would be virtually impossible to replicate such a long, intense effort in the lab.

Because individual reactions to the drug vary widely, Johnson said, caffeine is not for every athlete. A certified personal trainer, he once worked with a runner who could not even handle a cup of tea. Any performance benefit she might get would be outweighed by feeling extremely jittery. Other athletes, like Piampiano, get the jitters from caffeine when they are not racing, but have no problem on race days.

Johnson said caffeine is best used judiciously. "One of my pet peeves about caffeine ingestion is when you get to the dependence level," he said. "I have a little bit more of a public health overview of our use of caffeine in our nation. You find a lot of people who constantly ingest

caffeine throughout the day, and therefore at bedtime have trouble going to sleep and then need alcohol or some sort of sleep aid to get to
bed, and then in the morning are so groggy that they need caffeine
again, to get back into this kind of vicious cycle of supplementation.
And I think when you get to that stage, it's definitely a negative standpoint."

One of the awkward aspects of caffeine use is the fine line between
boosting your metabolism and doping. "The performance effects of it
have been proven," said Johnson. "So it is a performance-enhancing
substance, in some sense."

Many bike racers are enthusiastic caffeine users. One of the dominant
United States pro teams is sponsored by 5-hour Energy, and one of
the top Canadian pro teams is sponsored by Toronto's Jet Fuel Coffee.
Alison Dunlap, an American cyclist whose kudos include a mountain
bike world championship and national championships in mountain
biking and cyclocross, is emphatic about its benefits. "Caffeine is my
wonder drug. I take at least 100 to 200 milligrams in the latter part of
a race for a quick pick-me-up," she told *Bicycling* magazine. "Don't
caffeinate too early because once you start it's best not to stop or you'll
experience the crash when the caffeine wears off."

Some cyclists take caffeine to extremes. Alexi Grewal, the American cyclist who won a gold medal in the 1984 Olympics, used it constantly. "Rocket fuel was tea with one Vivarin, double rocket fuel was
tea with two," he wrote in an essay published in *VeloNews*. "As an amateur among the pros, caffeine injections replaced the pills and the
stomach cramps went away too."

While caffeine is a performance-enhancing drug, it's purely legal in
most cases. But it hasn't always been legal, and some cyclists have
crossed the line. Steve Hegg, an American cyclist who won gold and
silver medals in 1984, was disqualified from the 1988 Olympic team
after a urine test showed caffeine levels above the legal limit of twelve

micrograms per milliliter of urine. In 1994, world champion cyclist
Gianni Bugno was suspended from racing after a positive test for
caffeine—a urine sample showed 16.8 micrograms per milliliter (he
claimed he had ingested nothing more than coffee).

And it is not just cyclists who have been tripped up by caffeine.
American track star Inger Miller had to relinquish a bronze medal
she'd won in a sixty-meter event at the 1999 world indoor track championship, due to excessive caffeine use. Miller asserted that she'd had
only her usual morning coffee and a couple of Cokes after the event,
which was sponsored by Coca-Cola. "A cup of coffee is one thing, but
the small cups they served at the hotel, I don't know if that's a cup, a
half a cup. . . . It's difficult for me to say how much I had as far as micrograms [of caffeine] per liter," she told the Associated Press. "Who's
to say that I was legal when I was running the race and then the two
Cokes I drank that they provided me put me over the limit? I don't
know that. They don't know that. There's no way to re-create the situation, yet I'm the one held to high expectations."

While some athletic organizations still limit caffeine, as they do
other performance-enhancing substances, most now do not. Until
2004, the World Anti-Doping Agency and the International Olympic
Committee considered twelve micrograms per milliliter in urine to be
the maximum legal concentration. But they dropped caffeine from
their list of prohibited substances in 2004 because caffeine is so ubiq-
uitous that setting a threshold might lead athletes to be penalized for
what others would consider normal caffeine consumption. (An analysis of urine samples showed that caffeine use has not changed in the
wake of the rule change, probably because athletes can get optimal
performance-enhancing effects at much lower levels.)

The National Collegiate Athletic Association (NCAA) still has caffeine on its banned drug list, if urine concentrations exceed fifteen
micrograms per milliliter. To exceed the urine concentration, an athlete would likely have to consume more than ten milligrams of caffeine per kilo of body weight. Using the examples of eighty-kilo and

sixty-five-kilo athletes again, this would be more than ten SCADS and eight SCADS. But the urine tests are notoriously unreliable.

Even if it is legal to use caffeine in sports, is it ethical? As the Lance Armstrong doping scandal broke wide open in the fall of 2012, one young cyclist stated that caffeine had gotten a bit out of hand. Taylor Phinney—who had already represented the United States in two Olympics and won a stage in the Giro d'Italia by the age of twenty-two—said even with the increased awareness of and improved testing for performance-enhancing substances, bike culture is still too permissive. "There is widespread use of finish bottles, which are just bottles of crushed up caffeine pills and painkillers. That stuff can make you pretty loopy, and that is why I've never tried it. I don't even want to try it, as I feel it dangerous," Phinney said in an interview with *Velo-Nation*. So what does Phinney think is OK? He said he will use gels with caffeine and Coca-Cola, but not pills.

The effect of caffeine is the same, whether it is ingested in pills or coffee, but the perception is certainly different. The former seems like a drug; the latter, a popular beverage.

This is a distinction the American College of Sports Medicine makes, too, in a statement on caffeine and exercise: "For elite athletes, it is currently acceptable and reasonable to have their normal dietary coffee. However, if they deliberately take pure caffeine to gain an advantage on competitors, it is clearly unethical and is considered doping." By this definition many of the world's top endurance athletes would be considered dopers. But it's an ethical standard with no legal teeth.

Terry Graham, a professor at the University of Guelph, with decades of experience studying the physiology of caffeine metabolism, is a coauthor of that statement on doping. When I talked to him, he acknowledged that it is a gray area.

"It depends on your definition of doping," Graham told me. "If doping has to be illegal, then of course it is not doping. But if you are taking a substance which is not a critical nutrient, for the express purpose of getting an advantage over somebody else, then I would say it is doping."

Judging from the common strategic use of caffeine I saw at Kona, few agree with Graham's definition. Rather, they were quite open about using caffeine as a legal, effective performance-enhancing substance.

A secondary concern that affects cyclists, triathletes, and others who use caffeine to boost performance is the habit of relying on sleeping pills to help them rest at night. This is the "vicious cycle of supplementation" that Johnson mentioned. And it's a trap that any heavy caffeine user can fall into.

In Kona, I met a triathlete who said it is not unusual for them to take sleeping pills to wind down after an event. The practice sparked a controversy when England's soccer team took caffeine pills to amp up for an evening World Cup qualifying game in October 2012. But when the match was canceled, the players were left all amped up with no game to play. Some took sleeping pills to get a better night's rest. (Surprisingly, Graham told me that we metabolize caffeine at the same rate whether sitting at our desks or running marathons, so even if they had played a game, the soccer players would still have experienced postgame caffeination.) England played its delayed match with Poland the next day, and several sportswriters attributed the team's lackadaisical performance—they tied 1–1—to the sleeping pills.

Australian athletes, too, have fallen into this trap. After an Olympic swimmer acknowledged he had grown dependent on Stilnox (the sleeping aid known in the United States as Ambien), Australian authorities told their athletes competing in the London Olympics that they could not take sedatives. Australian Olympic Committee chief John Coates told Reuters, "We are very worried about the vicious cycle of athletes taking caffeine as a performance enhancer and then needing to take drugs such as Stilnox to get to sleep."

Coffee, pills, and energy gels are not the only caffeine delivery mechanisms that are common in elite sports. New products abound. Grinds Coffee Pouches, which are like packets of Skoal filled with coffee instead of tobacco, are catching on among Major League Baseball players. The caffeinated dip is now on hand in twelve clubhouses. And basketball star LeBron James is part owner of the company producing Sheets, a caffeinated product that dissolves on the tongue. "Taking a Sheet is part of my pregame and halftime ritual," James said in a press release. "I've tried tons of other products in the past and none compare. Sheets are a smart and convenient way to get energy."

And if you get amped up on Sheets for an evening game and have trouble sleeping, there are, believe it or not, Sleep Sheets. Hawked by tennis superstar Serena Williams, these gel strips are sleep aids that contain chamomile, melatonin, and theanine.

Back at Kona, the race that had started at dawn continued well past noon. It was early afternoon by the time Piampiano came running down Ali'i Drive, a third of the way into the marathon. A gentle breeze blew over the street from the beach, and surfers were riding the chest-high waves just offshore, but it was sweltering under the tropical sun along the road. Piampiano's red hair was pulled back in a ponytail, sunglasses obscured her blue eyes, and a visor shaded her determined face.

She had sixteen miles left to run, and she moved smartly, at a pace of 7:45 minutes per mile. Most of the race was behind her. She had already been racing for eight hours, with just two to go. This is the part of the race where fatigue—mental and physical—can utterly destroy an athlete. In her left hand, Piampiano clutched a little foil packet, a mocha energy gel that contained another fifty milligrams of caffeine.

After Piampiano ran by, I watched other triathletes as they passed through an aid station, greeted by volunteers shouting out, "water, water" and "energy gels, energy gels." The athletes danced through, stutter-stepping as they grabbed sponges to drizzle cool water on themselves, sipped water or Coke from paper cups, or grabbed Gu energy gels.

Gu was the first company to market energy gels in the United

States and is a longtime sponsor of the Ironman. The company specializes in producing single-serving, foil-packaged energy gels, designed to help athletes stayed fueled during endurance events. While in Kona, I met Gu Energy Labs founder and CEO Brian Vaughan. He told me that Gu gels combine carbohydrates with essential amino acids and electrolytes . . . and caffeine.

Vaughan said roughly two-thirds of his products are caffeinated and that athletes use the drug with great specificity. "The top-end athletes, the pros, want to be able to meter out caffeine during the course of an endurance event. At the beginning, perhaps, it's all decaf products. There's no problem with energy at the early stage of a race; a lot of adrenaline is going through the body. Toward the middle and end, athletes will look for different levels of caffeine. It's always nice to have that second wind late in the race, where you can energize the mind, stimulate the mind, with the central nervous system response from caffeine."

Vaughan said caffeine can enhance the mental focus that is so critical to endurance athletes, especially as fatigue sets in. "There are moments when the mind begins to wander; you become less competitive when you have these lapses," he told me. "To really be able to focus on smaller goals within the race is important for the competitive athlete."

Beyond blocking the sense of mental fatigue, caffeine has another significant effect on metabolism. For years, scientists thought that one of the drug's primary mechanisms was to spare the glycogen stored in muscles. The theory was that caffeine, by slightly increasing epinephrine (adrenaline), increased the level of free fatty acids in the blood, which muscles would use in lieu of stored glycogen.

"It's a beautiful theory," Terry Graham, the University of Guelph professor, told me. But his painstaking research has shown that it is simply wrong. "If you measure any aspect of metabolism during exercise with caffeine, you virtually never see a reflection of increased fat metabolism or decreased carbohydrate metabolism," he said. "And if you measure the glycogen levels, the data will vary because glycogen varies, but the majority will show no glycogen sparing."

Another Canadian researcher, who has previously collaborated with Graham, has taken a big step toward unlocking the mystery of caffeine's athletic enhancement. Mark Tarnopolsky is an Ontario physician and professor of pediatrics at McMaster University. He is also a national-class trail runner and competes internationally in winter triathlons, ski orienteering, and adventure racing. You might say he is uniquely qualified to understand caffeine in athletics.

When we spoke over the phone, he told me that one of the keys to muscular strength is found in the sarcoplasmic reticulum. This is essentially a bag of calcium inside a muscle. He said caffeine increases the amount of calcium released from the sarcoplasmic reticulum, and more calcium equals more force per muscular contraction.

To better understand this process, Tarnopolsky needed to test caffeine's effects on muscles without the interference of the brain. To do this, he clamped his subjects' legs into a force transducer, a device that measures the strength of a muscular effort. Then he electroshocked them.

This low-frequency electrical current was being delivered directly to the leg, mimicking the effort the muscles would make during a low-intensity run; therefore, the subjects' brains had no say over how strong the contraction would be. "I don't care how tired you are—if your wife left you that day, if you've lost every penny you ever owned—when that thing says go, it is going to drive that muscle," he said.

Tarnopolsky found greater force in the muscles of the subjects dosed with caffeine. "For a given input, your muscle gives you a slightly stronger contraction. So you can either run at the same speed with less input or run at a faster speed with the same input."

The caffeine effect at the muscular level is distinct from its mental effects. So caffeine has the potential to help endurance athletes in two very different ways, in different parts of the body. The drug blocks adenosine's "you are getting tired" mantra as it pours more coal on the intramuscular fires.

As a competitor, Tarnopolsky keeps his caffeine strategy pretty simple. An hour before a race, he usually drinks a large "Timmy's," as Canadians refer to a cup of coffee from their beloved Tim Hortons chain. That likely delivers about 150 milligrams of caffeine. During longer races he also uses caffeinated energy gels with about 50 milligrams of caffeine. In general, he shoots for about 2 milligrams per kilo of body weight.

⚡

While caffeine can seem like an athletic wonder drug, it is possible to overdo it. One dramatic case comes from a musher competing in the 1,050-mile Iditarod race between Anchorage and Nome, Alaska. In a 1978 paper, Dr. Verner Stillner recounted the epic exertions—and caffeine consumption—of a twenty-eight-year-old fisherman and trapper identified as Mr. A.

In the third week of the race, Mr. A. decided to mush for forty-eight hours straight. "Following an evening meal of pork chops, two cups of brewed coffee, and three cola drinks he resumed mushing in subzero temperatures with strong winds," Stillner wrote. "Despite this intake of an estimated 270–330 mg of caffeine with his meal, he experienced increasing difficulty staying awake. Two hours after the meal, he ingested 400 mg of caffeine (2 tablets of Vivarin, an over-the-counter preparation). Approximately 20 minutes later, he ingested an additional 400 mg. Thus, in less than 3 hours he had taken more than 1,000 mg of caffeine."

Mr. A. was used to moderate doses of caffeine—his daily intake averaged 270 to 360 milligrams—but few people can tolerate the massive dose he took that night. Not surprisingly, things became unpleasant as Mr. A., all jacked up on thirteen SCADs, followed his sled dogs into the frigid Alaskan darkness: "His hands became tremulous, and he experienced a pronounced buzzing in his ears. He perceived his miner's headlamp as emitting no more than a narrow band of light. The ascent of a long hill seemed as if 'it were a flat plain riddled with white stars.' Vertigo ensued, and he tumbled twice from his sled in a short interval. He experienced doubt as to whether he was really in a race and feared being alone."

But Mr. A. mushed through the night, his symptoms abating within six hours. He completed the race three days later. Dr. Stillner concluded, "As little as five 200-mg tablets of readily available over-the-counter preparations of caffeine appears sufficient to generate a delirium. Even smaller amounts may lead to sufficient sensory and motor disturbances to prove dangerous in situations such as long-distance driving. Such effects of caffeine merit closer attention."

In the end, Piampiano's race did not go as well as she had hoped. I watched her cross the finish line in just over ten hours. It was a fantastic time for a mortal—she beat 495 of the 524 elite women who'd qualified to race in Kona—but not for a professional triathlete. She theorized that her trouble might have been caused by cumulative fatigue from a long season.

Piampiano said the caffeine gels helped, especially when she started running the marathon. "I was turning to caffeine much earlier, overall, during the race than I would have normally," she said. "The caffeine was much appreciated, and I really noticed the difference in terms of having it. Without it, I would have completely just hit a wall and not been able to move forward."

The day after the race was, again, sunny and warm. Among the nineteen hundred triathletes prowling Kona, some were hobbling painfully, but not as many as you might expect. More notable were the many athletes who were spending their post–race day running or cycling, perhaps to loosen up their race-depleted legs.

And for those spectators who were couch potatoes but were so inspired by the triathlon that they dusted off an old ten-speed or laced up their running shoes? Caffeine helps them, too. A group of Australian researchers figured this out.

Their subjects were men who exercised less than an hour every week and did not regularly use much caffeine (less than 120 milligrams daily). They rode exercise bikes for thirty minutes, an hour after taking a gelatin capsule with either a placebo or a caffeine dose equivalent to 6 milligrams per kilogram. This is a hefty dose: five SCADS for a 140-pound man; seven SCADs for one who weighs 200. The results were unequivocal.

"This study demonstrated that a moderate dose of caffeine improved cycling performance in sedentary men," they reported. "Additionally, caffeine increased oxygen uptake and energy expenditure, without increased ratings of perceived exertion." In this case, it is the latter that's more important. The men did not feel that they were working any harder, but they burned more energy, and this could "motivate previously sedentary individuals to become more active, which in turn has positive effects on aerobic fitness and overall health."

But the researchers left off with one caveat: "Nonetheless, caffeine ingestion can be addictive with a variety of symptoms when withdrawal is attempted. Consequently, prescription of its use during exercise should be as a motivating tool during the initial stages of exercise only, particularly as the ergogenic effects of caffeine are partially diminished in habitual users."

They concisely synopsized the challenges of using caffeine well: It can motivate you and improve your performance, but it is also addicting. In other words, use it to train, use it to race, but use it judiciously.

CHAPTER 11

Joe for GIs

I t is easy to think of caffeine specifically, and our national obsession with stimulants more generally, as a recent phenomenon, but by now we know it's not. Consider this statement: "A chemical substance which stimulates brain, nerves, and muscles, is a daily necessity and is used by every single nation."

This comes not from the high-paced modern world, but from an era before cars, TVs, even radios—when horses clip-clopped down cobbled streets, people ambled to work, and things seemed to be altogether more civilized, at least through our nostalgic lenses. But caffeine was already popular, perhaps even essential in some situations. That sentence comes from the 1896 Report of the Secretary of War. And consider the next line. "When there is fatigue and the food is diminished such a stimulant is indispensable, and must be an ingredient of every reserve and emergency ration." More than a century ago, military leaders were trying to figure out how to keep soldiers amped up.

Some things have changed after a century of research on military stimulants. Notably, the first item listed in the report—extract of beef, in bouillon or tea—is no longer considered a stimulant. But the rest of the list will be familiar. There's kola nut, "a powerful and safe stimulant not accompanied by ill effects nor after depression. . . . It is now used to a very great extent by bicycle riders and by other people who undergo tiresome exertion." But kola nut is hard to keep fresh, the report concluded, and "impracticable in a reserve ration."

There is, of course, tea, which travels better than coffee. The report focused on compressed tea tablets. "One that is 1⅛ inches in diameter and three-eighths of an inch thick, weighing one-third of an ounce, is sufficient to make about 3-4 pints of strong tea. . . . These are excellent as an ingredient of the reserve ration, and probably better then coffee for the field. They are not recommended for emergency rations because the American soldier, with but few exceptions, wants coffee, and plenty of it." Not ideal for Americans, of course, but fine for our neighbors: "The tea tablets are now used by the Northwest Canadian mounted police and are entirely satisfactory, so far as known, but these people prefer tea to coffee."

And that brings us to coffee, which accounts for the bulk of the report on stimulants. "Coffee in liberal amounts should be a part of the emergency ration. Its valuable property in stimulating the mind, nerves and muscles is just what is needed in these times of great fatigue and deficient food."

And then, as now, we see that people were wrestling with the problem of how to get a delicious cup of fresh coffee in the field. "The berry will have to be roasted, for there will be no chance to do this in emergency cases, and roasted coffee, whether ground or not, will keep but a short period unless it is hermetically sealed." But the various cubes of compressed ground coffee were not good enough, their "aromatic substances" prone to evaporation. So the military enlisted the aid of Searle & Hereth, a Chicago pharmaceutical company. Searle had its own ideas about sealing the compressed coffee: "They have roasted and ground the coffee, compressed it into tablets, which were then sugar coated, hermetically sealing the contents." Unfortunately, the pharmacists' coffee tablets were too crumbly (Searle later had better success with other products like Dramamine, Metamucil, NutraSweet, and Enovid, an early oral contraceptive).

Extracts of coffee, too, proved of little use to the military in the late 1800s. The phrase "instant coffee" was not then in use, but this description of "solid extract of coffee" seemed to catch the essence of the soon-to-emerge market: "It made a very bad-tasted coffee, and it is presumed from the absence of such solid extracts from the market that their preparation involves the destruction of the aromatic and other substances, and that such articles are failures."

More than a century later, the U.S. military is still trying to figure out how best to caffeinate its soldiers. A handy result of this is that military scientists have conducted some of the most useful research on caffeine in general.

Some of that research is conducted at the Natick Soldier Research, Development and Engineering Center, half an hour west of Boston. It would look like a large suburban office park but for the soldiers standing guard at a gatehouse, complete with a blast barrier.

One of the buildings at Natick has a brightly lit room called the Warfighter Café. That's where Betty Davis, who leads the Performance Optimization Research Team, showed me a small table covered with snack foods—applesauce, beef jerky, energy bars, and nutritious "tube foods," which taste like pudding but come in a package that looks like a large tube of Crest. The products have two things in common. They are formulated for soldiers ("warfighters" in the current Department of Defense lexicon). And they all contain added caffeine.

Since 1962, the height of the Cold War, researchers at Natick have been developing products to improve conditions for soldiers in the field. There are even two large wind tunnels for testing gear in extreme conditions: One simulates tropical conditions; the other is a cold room, where temps can drop to minus seventy degrees Fahrenheit. The female-specific body armor developed here made *Time* magazine's list of Best Inventions of the Year 2012. This body armor represents what the researchers call "skin-out" work, which is anything to do with the exterior of a soldier's body. Davis works on the "skin-in" side of things: the soldier's physiology.

She showed me a plastic-wrapped ration, about the size of a small hardcover book. It's called a First Strike ration, a concentrated package of nutrition designed for soldiers moving quickly with minimal gear. Natick researchers developed it after studying how soldiers took apart their bulkier MRE (meals ready to eat) rations, stripping away the items they did not want.

"The MRE is the primary individual ration, and you get three per day," said Davis. "And in some cases, it is field stripped, because you need to have room for your ammo and things like that. So we did a survey asking what are you field stripping and why? And what we wanted to do with the First Strike ration is design a ration that provided the nutrition as well as give you that eat-on-the-move capability. It is considered an assault ration. So while the MRE provides about thirty-six hundred calories per day, this provides about twenty-nine hundred calories per day, so that's why it's called a restricted ration."

The idea is that soldiers can get a day's worth of sustenance from one First Strike ration instead of three MREs. Davis said that in order to compress the maximum nutrition into one small package that is about half the size and weight of three MREs, all of the foods in the package are specially formulated. "The components in here we would fortify with certain things, one of which is caffeine for alertness, extra carbohydrates for energy, as well as protein for muscle wasting," she said.

The First Strike rations include plenty of caffeine. For starters, there is Stay Alert gum, with five pieces per pack, each piece containing 100 milligrams, a bit more than a SCAD. This was originally developed by a subsidiary of Wrigley, working with researchers at the Walter Reed Army Institute of Research. The gum was tested at Natick. And there is Zapplesauce, caffeinated applesauce. It comes in a plastic pouch and packs 110 milligrams of caffeine. There is a mocha-flavored First Strike Nutritious Energy Bar, also packing 110 milligrams of caffeine. Some of the rations also include instant coffee (which soldiers sometimes put between their cheek and gum, like a dip of Skoal, a sort of do-it-yourself version of the Grinds Coffee Pouches) or caffeinated mints.

In a little bowl on the table, Davis had a pile of caffeinated meat sticks that looked like Slim Jims, sliced into two-inch lengths. As I chewed on one, which was delicious, a fair-haired man with an unassuming manner walked in and asked, "Are they feeding you already?" This was Harris Lieberman, a psychologist with the U.S. Army Research Institute of Environmental Medicine, also at Natick. Lieberman, who has studied the drug for three decades, has an encyclopedic knowledge of caffeine. In fact, he has written encyclopedia entries on caffeine. And he understands its advantages for soldiers.

He tried a piece of the beef jerky. "It's really good," he said, "and it really does completely mask the caffeine."

Caffeine's naturally bitter flavor presented a challenge when developing the Stay Alert gum. "The formulation is not optimized the way a gum is normally optimized to get the sustained flavor and the pleasurable flavor," he said. "The whole point of the flavor is that you don't have this very bitter flavor when you start chewing."

While the flavoring was a challenge, the gum has a big advantage over more traditional caffeine delivery mechanisms: The caffeine tends to be absorbed sublingually in the mucous membranes. Scientists at Walter Reed Army Institute of Research found that the caffeinated kick of gum takes full effect within five to ten minutes, as opposed to thirty to forty-five minutes for caffeine ingested in a pill or a beverage like coffee or cola.

The gum research became a minor political issue when Illinois Republican representative Dennis Hastert added $250,000 in research funds to a 1998 federal defense spending bill, allowing the Wrigley subsidiary Amurol to study possible military applications for caffeinated gum, and another congressman criticized the budget add-on as a bit of pork for a hometown business. Wrigley later licensed its patented caffeinated-gum technology to the company that produced Stay

Alert gum for the military. (In 2004, when a pair of New Jersey entrepreneurs began marketing caffeinated gum under the Jolt brand, Wrigley sued, claiming patent infringement, even though it was not then marketing a caffeinated gum. But Wrigley's caffeinated gum would become far more controversial by 2013.)

Lieberman said products that offer such rapid delivery of caffeine have applications beyond the military. "Just to give you an example from the civilian sector, if you're driving and you become sleepy suddenly, you want to be able to quickly fix that problem," he said. "You don't want to wait for the caffeine to start working. You want to get the effect as immediately as you possibly can, before you have an accident. And certainly there are a lot of potential military applications, where you need to solve the problem immediately. So that's a definite advantage of the product over more conventional caffeine-containing products. Minutes can make a difference in these situations."

Lieberman pointed out the tubes on the table. One of the silvery vessels was labeled "Caffeinated Apple Pie"; the other, "Caffeinated Chocolate Pudding." The pie is boosted with one hundred milligrams of caffeine; the pudding with two hundred milligrams. These are products made especially for pilots who fly U-2 spy planes at altitudes reaching seventy thousand feet. Lieberman walked over to a shelf in the café and showed me the sort of helmet the pilots wear.

"They have a special delivery system, because they are encapsulated like a spaceman," he said. "The U-2 airplane is a reconnaissance airplane that flies incredibly high, and it's not pressurized, so therefore the pilots have to wear a pressure suit and a helmet. They go on fairly long missions. Not superlong, but a lot longer than you'd want to be up there without anything to eat or drink. The only way they can get things into their mouth is through this little gizmo here." The gizmo he was referring to is a sort of glorified straw that allows them to slurp down the tube food.

Lieberman is quite familiar with this system. He and his colleagues once used it to study caffeine's effects on flying skills. The subjects were twelve U.S. Air Force pilots, who were tested at night on flight simulators. They also completed mood surveys, a symptom questionnaire, and tests on cognitive tasks. The study was unique in looking at caffeinated food, as opposed to caffeinated beverages or pills.

They found that caffeine helped, and delivering it in a food, as opposed to a beverage or pill, worked fine. And instead of having to take food and caffeine separately, fumbling each time with the food tube, the pilots could get both at once. "Based on the results from this investigation, caffeinated tube food is an effective tool for sustaining cognitive performance and vigilance during extended and nighttime food operations," the researchers wrote. "Results may also be generalized to other populations who wear complex protective clothing, such as chemical warfare-protective or spacesuits, for extended work periods."

Lieberman has also studied caffeine's effects on military personnel on the ground . . . and in the water. For one of his experiments, he studied an elite subset of soldiers in an extremely intense situation.

The Navy SEAL special forces teams have long been known as some of America's ultimate soldiers. Their reputation was further burnished when they led the 2011 raid that killed Osama bin Laden. But the SEALs—whose name is compressed from "sea, air, land"—do not take all comers. You have to try out. And the toughest period of SEAL training is known as Hell Week, a brutal initiation on the beaches near San Diego.

Here's how Lieberman described Hell Week in a 2002 paper:

> The challenges of Hell Week include a variety of activities such as surf immersion, where students, arms linked, sit in a line so the surf strikes them in the face. This lasts for a period of 10–20 min depending upon water temperature. Boat push ups are another frequent activity with trainees expected to raise inflatable boats over their heads, and then as a team push them up until their arms are fully extended. The boats contain life vests, paddles, and often

a considerable amount of water. Other more traditional forms of physical training such as push-ups and sit-ups are frequently required of trainees by the instructors. Psychological stressors include verbal confrontations with instructors and activities with no-win outcomes. During Hell Week trainees only have a few hours to sleep during irregular breaks in training and are often wet and cold. . . . Generally, more than one-half the trainees who start Hell Week do not complete it and therefore cannot continue SEAL training.

Those who just cannot go on have the DOR (drop-on-request) option—they simply walk over to a shiny brass bell, ring it, and they are done, their SEAL career over before it has begun. In all, it is truly a hellish experience. And there is yet another diabolical aspect to the week of torture: The aspiring SEALs are not allowed any caffeine . . . except for the purposes of science.

In this extreme event that pushes strong men to their limits, Lieberman saw an opportunity to assess the effectiveness of caffeine on sleep-deprived, highly stressed soldiers. Ninety subjects volunteered for his study; just sixty-eight completed it (the rest had chosen to ring the bell). The men averaged twenty-four years old with three years in the military. After seventy-two hours with almost no sleep, they were given capsules containing 100, 200, or 300 milligrams of caffeine, or identical placebos.

The recruits then took a variety of tests, including a series of cognitive tests on laptop computers. One involved detecting a faint, infrequent visual stimulus. Another combined short-term learning and motor skills by requiring the recruits to learn a random sequence of twelve keystrokes. They recorded their moods and perceptions of sleepiness. And they took a marksmanship test with a laser mounted on a disabled AK-47.

The results were unequivocal. Caffeine significantly improved the subjects' performance on all the tests except marksmanship, which was unaffected by the drug.

Lieberman concluded, "Even in the most adverse circumstances, moderate doses of caffeine can improve cognitive function, including vigilance, learning memory, and mood state. When cognitive performance is critical and must be maintained during exposure to severe stress, administration of caffeine may provide a significant advantage. A dose of 200 mg appears to be optimal under such conditions."

When we discussed caffeine in his office, in another building on the Natick campus, Lieberman told me that caffeine boosts can help civilians, too. "Under most conditions, caffeine will improve your ability to attend to relatively infrequent, but potentially very important, stimuli," said Lieberman. He said this is a potentially lifesaving benefit equally applicable to a soldier on watch or a civilian on a long drive on a lonely highway.

"If you are going to use it, you should use it moderately," he said. "There's a lot of disagreement among scientists about whether caffeine is a beneficial compound or something which we should be more concerned about its negative effects than its positive effects. So there's no real absolute scientific consensus, and as long as there's scientific controversy, I think it's appropriate that the public be aware of the pros and cons and make their own decision."

Making decisions about caffeine use is complicated by the challenges of quantifying doses, given the variable caffeine levels in coffee and tea. Lieberman said, "It's very hard to do the math. But I think individuals tend to be pretty sensitive to the level of caffeine they are taking. Because if they take too much caffeine, they are probably going to get some adverse changes in how they are feeling."

Frank Ritter, of the Applied Cognitive Science Lab at Penn State, was conducting caffeine research supported by the Office of Naval Research when he became intrigued by the question of how best to quantify caffeine consumption. He believes that even caffeine-savvy people often do not understand just how much caffeine they have taken. As a follow-up to his naval research, he developed a mobile phone app for civilian and military use alike.

Caffeine Zone allows you to enter your caffeine consumption at any time—a sixteen-ounce cup of coffee, for example, or a stick of Stay Alert gum—and see a graph showing just how much caffeine you have in your system. If you want to optimize your metabolism, you can set limits and your phone will alert you when your levels are too high or too low or when it is time to dial it back in order to sleep well. By June 2013, nearly eighty thousand people had downloaded the app.

Many other researchers have considered caffeine's military applications. A paper from NASA's Ames Research Center looked at the effectiveness of caffeine in preparing sailors on aircraft carriers for four-day surge operations (SURGEOPs). The authors suggest saving caffeine's kick for when it is most needed:

> Shipboard environments are famous for heavy caffeine consumption. To enhance caffeine's effects in regular users, crewmembers should be encouraged to cut back significantly on caffeine (but not stop its use) for at least two days before the SURGEOP (preferably a week) and avoid caffeine until 18–20 hr into it. Certainly by two days before the start of the SURGEOP caffeine consumption should have been reduced by half.
>
> Caffeine should then be used strategically, starting in the late night/early morning hours (0100–0300) and tapered as morning approaches (0800). Caffeine takes about 30 min to have an effect (peak plasma levels occur in 30–60 min) and its stimulant effects last for about 3–4 hr (half-life is about 3–7 hr). Some caffeine may be necessary again in the mid afternoon to counter the mid afternoon dip in alertness that occurs whether or not lunch was eaten. Caffeine should not be taken during relatively alert periods nor within several hours of sleep onset, although this may not be a problem in a surge operation in which sleep onset is delayed 30+ hr.

This is a fairly specific caffeine prescription for a four-day naval cruise. It is more applicable to sailors than to civilians, but you might want to refer back to it should you suddenly have to drive alone from Miami to Seattle in four days.

It is not just shipboard environments that are famous for heavy caffeine use. Caffeine consumption is high on military bases—energy drinks are abundant. Army researcher Robin Toblin and her colleagues found that 45 percent of U.S. Army and Marine service members in combat platoons deployed to Operation Enduring Freedom in Afghanistan in 2010 drank at least one energy drink daily. Fourteen percent drank three or more. And they found an association between energy drink use and sleep.

"Service members drinking three or more energy drinks a day were significantly more likely to report sleeping <4 hours a night on average than those consuming two drinks or fewer," Toblin wrote. "Those who drank three or more drinks a day also were more likely to report sleep disruption related to stress and illness and were more likely to fall asleep during briefings or on guard duty."

The study could not attribute the cause of the sleepiness to energy drinks, but only show the association. And the authors did not quantify the caffeine the service members consumed, either from energy drinks or from other sources. Still, the study prompted a word of caution in an accompanying editorial note: "Service members should be educated that the long-term health effects of energy drink use are unknown, that consuming high doses of energy drinks might affect mission performance and sleep, and that, if used, energy drinks should be consumed in moderation."

⚡

Scott Killgore is an expert on sleep and caffeine use in the military. When I met the neuropsychologist, he was sitting at a sort of cockpit before three large computer monitors in his office with a view over the leafy lawn of McLean Hospital in Belmont, Massachusetts. He is trim and fit, and his erect posture and short hair reflect his military background. Killgore's early research was on brain activation in adolescents during emotional processing, and he might not have started studying caffeine at all if not for the terrorist attacks in 2001.

"I went in the army after the September eleventh attacks happened," he told me. "I just sort of started reevaluating where my life was at that point and thought, 'I want to contribute.'" When he went on active duty, Killgore was assigned to a lab where researchers were studying the effects of chronic sleep deprivation. He is so interested in sleep cycles that he wears a special device that looks like a beefed-up wristwatch. It detects your movements at night. Upload the data to a computer and it will display a chart that can tell you how rested you are.

Killgore spent five years on active duty, trying to understand how to help soldiers serve under the stresses of combat, especially through the use of caffeine. He said soldiers face contradictory threats. On one hand, there is the possibility of a surprise attack of deadly force. On the other, the draining tugs of boredom and exhaustion.

"In the military, quite often you find yourself in situations where you are changing time zones or you need to stay up all night to do a watch, and there may be times when you are not able to get the amount of sleep that you need," he said. "And during those times, a person may need to take some kind of a caffeinated supplement, like a caffeinated gum, that might help you to stay alert and awake and vigilant. A lot of times military watch may be very boring, but one critical incident may be a life-or-death incident, and you need to stay awake and alert during that time."

This tension between boredom and danger is analogous to other situations. In a way, it is like firefighters zoning out before the TV at a station house, then suddenly having to respond to a four-alarm fire. Or a policeman in the drowsy hours of an uneventful night shift unexpectedly confronted with an armed and violent criminal. Or an ER doctor rising from a snooze to treat a newly admitted accident victim. Less dramatic, but just as much a life-or-death situation, is a long-haul trucker pulling into Los Angeles at two a.m. on the ragged edge of a three-day run. And caffeine has other benefits that are not so apparent.

In one study, Killgore and his colleagues at Walter Reed looked at twenty-five active-duty military subjects. The subjects were not allowed to sleep for three nights, while they received either caffeinated gum or a placebo, administered in double-blind conditions. The caffeine group got two hundred milligrams of caffeine every two hours, in four doses.

To study the drug's effect on risk-taking behavior, Killgore used a Balloon Analog Risk Test (BART). In essence, the subjects used laptops that displayed a balloon. If they pumped up the balloon until it was pretty big but did not pop, they would get a cash reward. If the balloon popped, no cash.

Killgore wrote, "Overall, after three nights without sleep, those receiving caffeine were popping fewer balloons and taking home more money than those receiving placebo, suggesting that caffeine was protective against behaviorally measured impairments in risk-related judgment and impulsiveness during prolonged sleep deprivation."

It might be hard to imagine the direct civilian application for these findings, unless you are a high-stakes gambler on a three-day poker jag. But the study is another indication of the breadth of caffeine's effects. Killgore speculates that the results probably come from caffeine activating the prefrontal cortex, the region of the brain that is critical for so-called executive function, such as high-level problem solving.

Taking advantage of caffeine is all about moderation, Killgore said. "I think judicious use of caffeine is probably the way to go about it, rather than just drinking it without any consideration for the time of day or for how much you had during the day. That can lead to a lot of problems with sleep and make you feel anxious and jittery and have a lot of bad side effects."

Killgore said that plenty of research frontiers remain to be explored. "We don't really know the effects that caffeine may have on priming the brain, in a sense, for a possible traumatic event. Could that increased arousal have an effect on being exposed to some type of traumatic event and change the way that you encode that information? Could it maybe change the way you respond to that event and predispose you to PTSD? We really don't know at this point. The research hasn't been done. I think it's a reasonable one to look at with research, to try to understand the effect caffeine may have on preparing the brain to respond in a more anxious way."

These questions of caffeine's effects on sleep and on anxiety have occupied researchers for decades. And some of their findings put the white powder in a shadowy light, if not a black hat.

CHAPTER 12

Insomnia, Anxiety, and Panic

Amy Wolfson knows sleep. An energetic woman with short, curly brown hair, the professor of psychology at the College of the Holy Cross serves on the board of the National Sleep Foundation, is the author of *The Woman's Book of Sleep*, and has spent much of her career studying sleep. When I met her in her office on the verdant campus on a hill overlooking Worcester, Massachusetts, she told me sleep is undervalued in American culture. "We spend at least a third of our lives asleep," she said, "but often we don't get enough sleep, and I'm interested in the ramifications of that."

Sleep disruption is a well-known side effect of caffeine use, but it is highly variable. Some people can drink coffee until the moment they turn in and sleep like babies. Others need to stop drinking caffeine by noon, or they will lie abed, gnashing their teeth, hearts thumping in their chests, thoughts racing. This brings us back to one of caffeine's conundrums: It is a fantastic drug for treating the symptom of sleepiness, but it can lead to increased sleepiness by interfering with sleep.

"Sleep researchers have been . . . I would almost use the word 'guilty,' of sometimes giving a confused message with regard to caffeine," Wolfson told me. "Caffeine is sometimes recommended as a sleep countermeasure, recommended for the military, recommended for pilots, recommended for train drivers, et cetera. I have colleagues that have devoted their careers to looking at countermeasures to sleepiness that aren't sleep.

"And then at the same time, you have the insomnia researchers that have for decades said, 'Oh, caffeine is a bad thing. For three to five hours before you are going to try to fall asleep, make sure you have caffeine out of your system.' For individuals who suffer from insomnia, they are given lectures in cognitive behavioral treatment programs to stay away from caffeine. So we have had a kind of love-hate relationship with caffeine. At least in the field of sleep research."

Wolfson told me she is especially interested in adolescents' caffeine use and the relationship between caffeine and a population of sleepy teens, which researchers are starting to scrutinize. In 2006, Maryland researchers found an association between caffeine use and adolescents who have trouble sleeping and feel tired in the morning. Wolfson and a colleague found a similar trend when they surveyed high school students about caffeine use. The students in a high-caffeine group—who took caffeine from coffee, energy drinks, and sodas—reported more daytime sleepiness, expected more energy enhancement from caffeine, and said they used it to get through the day.

Looking at younger caffeine consumers, a team of Nebraska researchers surveyed 228 parents and found that their five- to seven-year-old children drank approximately 52 milligrams of caffeine daily, and eight- to twelve-year-old children drank 109 milligrams daily. Those children who used the most caffeine slept fewer hours.

Wolfson believes the emergence of the new generation of energy drinks is related to a population of sleepy teens, and that excessive caffeine use by young people is part of a larger problem.

"I don't think that every person who stops at Starbucks on their way to work or Dunkin' Donuts, or, as we do in my house, brew our Peet's Coffee every morning, is necessarily sleep deprived," she said. "But there may be a group that is getting an inadequate amount of sleep, and probably a higher percentage of adolescents than adults, who are going to be at risk for gravitating toward those products."

Caffeine's sleep-disrupting properties are so reliable that researchers sometimes use it to induce insomnia in healthy subjects. And it does not take a whopping dose to affect sleep. Swiss scientist Hans-Peter Landolt used an electroencephalogram to measure brain wave activity in healthy subjects who took two hundred milligrams of caffeine (less than three SCADs) in the morning. By that night's bedtime, the morning caffeine was still affecting the subjects. The effects were small, and not severely sleep disruptive, but they were there. Bedtime reactions to caffeine may also hinge on stress—among people who are not insomniacs, caffeine has a stronger effect on those who are vulnerable to stress-induced sleep disturbance.

A team of California scientists found another variable in how caffeine affects sleep: chronotype. That term describes our time-of-day preferences. Some of us are morning people, often known as larks, while others are evening people, better known as owls. In a study of fifty university students consuming caffeine at will, who used wrist-activated motion detectors and sleep logs, the scientists found that morning people were most susceptible to caffeine's sleep-disrupting effects. They noted that the findings were limited by the group—all university students, mostly sleep deprived, and with relatively few morning people among them. Still, their 2012 paper was the first to report a possible association between chronotype and caffeine's effects on sleep quality, suggesting there is plenty of room for more research.

Even though virtually all of us are aware of caffeine's effects on sleep, we often don't fully appreciate them. That is the message from a 2008 review of caffeine and daytime sleepiness. Authors Timothy Roehrs and Thomas Roth said that caffeine does not affect REM sleep, as other stimulants do, but decreases stages three and four sleep, which account for about 20 percent of our sleeping time and include some of our most restful, restorative sleep. "The risks to sleep and alertness of regular caffeine use are greatly underestimated by both the general population and physicians," they concluded. Again, there's that caffeine conundrum—should we use it to fight daytime fatigue or do without and see if our energy levels improve?

⚡

Sleeplessness can be troubling, but it's usually not debilitating. But caffeine can have more significant effects on the minds of those of us who are susceptible to it, by triggering anxiety. Anxiety itself is remarkably common. In any given year, forty million American adults will suffer from clinically significant anxiety, making it the most prevalent form of psychiatric disorder.

John Greden, of the University of Michigan, has written extensively on the link between caffeine and anxiety. He noted that while some people are more susceptible, too much caffeine can make almost anyone anxious. In a 1974 paper, "Anxiety or Caffeinism: A Diagnostic Dilemma," he wrote, "Relevant to this endeavor is the overlooked fact that high doses of caffeine—or 'caffeinism'—can produce pharmacological actions that cause symptoms essentially indistinguishable from those of anxiety neuroses."

Greden highlighted three cases he encountered while working at Walter Reed Army Medical Center. The first was a twenty-seven-year-old nurse who complained of lightheadedness, tremulousness, breathlessness, headache, and irregular heartbeat. She was first diagnosed with an anxiety reaction, related to her fear that her husband might be deployed to Vietnam. She was skeptical of this diagnosis, and after searching for a dietary cause, she figured it might be coffee.

The nurse was able to trace her symptoms to when she bought a fresh-drip coffee pot. "Because this coffee was 'so much better,' she had begun consuming an average of 10 to 12 cups of strong black coffee a day—more than 1,000 mg of caffeine," Greden wrote. In this case, the cure was simple. Once she withdrew from coffee, nearly all of her symptoms vanished. For one week she was tired, then felt better and said she was "truly awake in the morning for the first time in years."

Another subject, an "ambitious 37-year-old Army lieutenant colonel," presented with chronic anxiety. He also complained of insomnia and loose stools. He drank eight to fourteen cups of coffee daily, plus three or four colas, and hot cocoa at bedtime. But he was unwilling to accept his diagnosis and "responded with incredulous cynicism" when informed that caffeine could be causing the problems. When the officer finally reduced his caffeine intake, his symptoms improved dramatically.

The last subject, a thirty-four-year-old army personnel sergeant who bragged of being "the first one in the office in the morning and the last one to go at night," presented with recurrent headaches. Tests showed significantly elevated anxiety levels. Greden wrote, "When questioned about his caffeine use he responded as if it were a reflection of his masculinity: 'I can easily put away 10 to 15 cups a day, I drink more coffee than anyone else in my office.'" Adding up his coffee, tea, cola, and headache medication, Greden calculated the patient consumed approximately fifteen hundred milligrams daily. This is a massive dose, equal to twenty SCADs. As with the others, when the patient reduced his caffeine consumption, his symptoms were almost completely alleviated.

Clearly, these are extreme examples. Most Americans top out at three or four cups of coffee daily. But they illustrate an important point. "From the clinical perspective, many individuals complaining of anxiety will continue to receive substantial benefit from psychopharmacological agents," Greden wrote. "For an undetermined number of others, subtracting one drug—caffeine—may be of greater benefit than adding another." So the ideal first-line treatment for anxiety in a patient who uses caffeine is to eliminate the caffeine and see how the patient responds, before prescribing antianxiety medication.

Greden later looked at how anxiety affects caffeine consumption. In a 1985 paper he noted that caffeine might contribute to anxiety in normal adults or psychiatric inpatients, but it is not likely a contributing factor for many patients with anxiety disorder. That is because "high anxiety appears to deter anxious individuals from high caffeine consumption."

So while high levels of caffeine make most people anxious, patients who suffer from anxiety disorder have probably figured this out and avoid the drug. Presciently, Greden left off with these words: "Caffeine should provide a pharmacological probe with which to study further the pathophysiology of panic and other anxiety disorders."

It also appears that habitual caffeine consumption may inure us to its anxiety-producing effects. In a study of more than four hundred people, looking at alertness, anxiety, and headache before and after they took 250 milligrams of caffeine (in two doses, ninety minutes apart) or a placebo, Peter Rogers found that even the subjects with a genetic predisposition to caffeine-induced anxiety developed tolerance to this effect, even if their regular daily consumption averaged just 128 milligrams, less than two SCADs.

⚡

All of caffeine's effects—from athletic and cognitive boosts to sleeplessness and anxiety—vary, depending on how quickly we process the drug. The half-life of caffeine in the human body is about four or five hours. That is the time it will take for the caffeine concentration to drop 50 percent. But this can be dramatically different from person to person. For women on birth control pills, it is twice as long; they will get double the kick from the same amount of caffeine. (Pregnant women, especially those in the last four weeks of their term, see this effect even more strongly. However, many women forego caffeine in pregnancy and would not experience this.) Smokers process caffeine twice as quickly; they will get half the caffeine kick as a nonsmoker. The effect also varies with body weight.

To understand these variables, it helps to imagine a couple. The man is a smoker who weighs 180 pounds. The woman is on birth control and weighs 135 pounds. If they sit down for a cup of coffee, she will get a caffeine effect that is nearly five times stronger—he will need five cups of coffee to equal her one. This is what I call the *Mad Men* Meets *Sex and the City* Effect.

I use *Mad Men* because people smoked like chimneys in the era glorified in that show. But American smoking rates have plummeted since, from just over 40 percent to just under 20 percent. Nonsmokers need half as much caffeine to get the same kick. *Sex and the City* applies to the 17 percent of American women taking birth control pills—they, too, need half as much caffeine to get the same kick. Both trends— fewer cigarettes and more birth control pills—have the effect of making every milligram of caffeine go a little further.

The decline in coffee consumption has tracked with the decline in smoking and the rise in oral contraception. Although these lifestyle changes are not the primary cause of the decline in coffee drinking (there is no dearth of smoking guns), it is intriguing to think they might play a small role.

The mechanism at work in smokers and people on oral contraceptives is something called cytochrome P450 1A2, also known as CYP1A2. This is the primary enzyme we use to break down caffeine into its metabolites, accounting for some of the variability in how we metabolize caffeine (its cousin CYP2E1 also plays a role). The enzymes essentially reverse the last step that chemical companies take in manufacturing caffeine; they demethylate it into its metabolites, mostly paraxanthine (which also has caffeine-like effects), theobromine, and theophylline.

Pregnancy, oral contraceptives, and liver disease inhibit the enzyme, while smoking increases it. Strangely, vegetables in your diet can also play a role—cruciferous vegetables like broccoli can increase the enzyme activity, while apiaceous vegetables such as celery can reduce it. (Making things even more complex, women get a stronger enzyme response from the cruciferous vegetables than do men.)

In addition to the other variables in how we metabolize caffeine— including our size, acquired tolerance, smoking habits, use of oral contraceptives, and the amount of broccoli we put down—scientists are constantly learning more about how genetics influences the way we metabolize caffeine.

In a 2010 literature review, Amy Yang, of the University of Chicago, used twin studies to better understand the genetic basis of caffeine metabolism. Her review found that there is a strong genetic predisposition to caffeine preference and an especially strong genetic influence among those who use caffeine heavily (more than five cups of coffee per day in one study; greater than 625 milligrams daily in another). Yang also noted that genetics accounts for two of the best-known side effects of caffeine use. "Laboratory studies in human subjects show that susceptibility of some individuals to certain effects such as anxiety and insomnia can be accounted for by specific alleles of the [adenosine] receptors."

Being able to pin down a genetic aspect of sleep disruption helps to fill in a picture first sketched in preparation for the Chattanooga Coca-Cola trial. Writing in the journal *Sleep*, Hans-Peter Landolt noted that Harry Hollingworth had observed a few subjects who had no trouble sleeping after small doses of caffeine. Now, Landolt said, we can start to see the mechanisms that cause such variations. "One century after Hollingworth," he wrote, "pharmacogenetic studies of caffeine not only reveal insights into a distinct molecular contribution to individual caffeine sensitivity, but also indicate that A2A receptors are part of a biological pathway that regulates sleep in mammals."

Of the four types of adenosine receptors, two play leading roles. A1 receptors are the most widespread adenosine receptors in the human brain and are abundant in the cortex (cortical neurons are important for higher cognitive function). The A2A receptors Landolt refers to are more confined to areas deeper in the brain, in the basal ganglia, where they are involved with movement, motor learning, motivation, and reward.

Some people inherit a genetic trait that affects the way they metabolize caffeine. Specific individual genetic variants are known as single-nucleotide polymorphisms. That's a mouthful, so it is easy to see why scientists simply call them SNPs (pronounced SNIP). A gene known as ADORA2A regulates the A2A receptors. People who have a variant of this gene are far more susceptible to caffeine's effects. Yang wrote that one of these SNPs has outsize importance in caffeine-related psychiatric disorders: "The finding that the same SNP is associated with both caffeine-induced anxiety and panic disorder supports the observation that panic disorder patients are particularly susceptible to caffeine-induced anxiety and suggests that polymorphisms in the A2A receptor may influence both."

Regarding panic disorder, Yang is referring to research by the Brazilian doctor Antonio Nardi and his colleagues. Nardi was trying to better understand the mechanisms of panic attacks, using caffeine, as Greden had suggested, as a "pharmacological probe."

People who suffer from panic disorder have repeated, sudden panic attacks in which they feel they are losing control and that something horrible is happening. The attacks are transient, but they can be utterly debilitating. Often, the person will fear he or she is having a heart attack or is about to die. Panic attacks are remarkably common worldwide, afflicting about fifteen people out of every one thousand, and are twice as common among women.

For a study published in 2007, Nardi looked at three distinct groups of subjects. The control group comprised healthy people with no history of panic disorder. The second group included people with a history of panic disorder. The third group comprised first-degree relatives of the panic disorder group—parents, siblings, or children—who had no history of panic attacks.

Nardi gave all the subjects coffee or decaf made from instant Brazilian coffee. The caffeine content in the caffeinated coffee was high—480 milligrams per fifteen ounces (it likely included those caffeine-rich robusta beans). This would be equivalent to six Red Bulls, about forty ounces of moderately strong coffee, or twenty-four ounces of Starbucks coffee—more than six SCADs.

None of Nardi's subjects had panic attacks or increased anxiety after drinking the decaf. But 52 percent of the panic disorder patients suffered a panic attack after drinking the caffeinated coffee, while none of the control subjects did.

The unexpected finding was this: 41 percent of the first-degree relatives of the panic disorder patients also suffered panic attacks. These were people who had no history of panic attacks, and yet one strong dose of caffeine induced an attack.

In another study, Nardi fine-tuned the test. This time, he used the same 480-milligram caffeine challenge on four groups. In addition to a control group and a panic disorder group, he studied subjects with one of two types of common anxiety. One group had what is known as generalized social anxiety disorder (GSAD). This is a condition characterized by the fear of most social situations. The other group had performance social anxiety disorder (PSAD), which typically involves the fear of speaking, eating, or writing in public.

The results were similar to those in the first study. Nobody experienced a panic attack after drinking decaf, none of the control group ever experienced a panic attack, and 61 percent of the panic disorder patients experienced a panic attack after drinking the strongly caffeinated coffee.

The new information came from the two subgroups of anxiety disorder. The performance social anxiety patients had more panic attacks after drinking caffeine than the generalized social anxiety patients— a lot more. Fifty-three percent of the former subgroup had panic attacks triggered by caffeine, versus 16 percent in the latter.

Nardi wrote that his research suggests the performance social anxiety disorder is biologically different than generalized social anxiety disorder and closer to panic disorder. Interestingly, it's a distinction clarified by caffeine.

⚡

Nardi was not the first to challenge panic disorder patients with caffeine. In other studies, they have illuminated hidden corners of the caffeinated brain.

In a 1993 letter to *The American Journal of Psychiatry*, three New York doctors wrote, "In the course of a study of the effects of caffeine infusion in sleeping panic disorder patients, generalized anxiety disorder patients, and healthy comparison subjects, we have observed the onset of olfactory hallucinations, promptly after infusion, in two of seven patients."

So, yes, this is a bit weird. First of all, the subjects were sound asleep when the researchers injected them with 250 milligrams of caffeine—four SCADs, or about as much as a twelve-ounce cup of Starbucks coffee or four Red Bulls.

One of the subjects, with no history of psychiatric disorder, woke up fourteen minutes after the injection. That is not surprising. Nor is it surprising that he felt shaky, and had rapid breathing and heartbeat—he'd been mainlining caffeine. What was surprising was that he reported an "interesting smell or taste—more like a smell."

This was the olfactory hallucination—sensing a smell that did not exist. And he was not alone. Another subject, with generalized anxiety disorder, awakened three minutes after the injection, "experiencing a smell like that of plastic or burnt coffee."

Curiously, yet another subject, who did have a history of panic disorder, experienced hallucinations including "dancing visual patterns and an undescribed sound."

Apparently, these three subjects got off light, getting ripped from their dreams by a mere 250 milligrams; another subject got a 500-milligram injection, also while sound asleep (which may have been unpleasant, but did not induce hallucinations). The doctors concluded, "The observations here suggest that further study of the adenosine system may add to our understanding of hallucination formation."

A case stranger still was reported in 2007 by a team of Greek researchers. Studying a thirty-one-year-old male with panic disorder, they gave him a 400-milligram caffeine challenge. The caffeine precipitated a panic attack, "characterized by severe anxiety, intense fear, jitteriness, accelerated heart rate, sweating, chest pain, dizziness, fear of fainting and/or dying, and an urge to escape from the experimental setting." That is a textbook description of a panic attack, not surprising after taking 400 milligrams of caffeine. The unexpected finding was the strange sensation that came just before the panic attack: "He reported a special type of auditory hallucination: he could hear vividly and repeatedly, in an echo-form, the last words of each thought he had. According to the patient's report, these hallucinations emerged suddenly—while he was in a state of minimal-to-moderate anxiety— and certainly *preceded* the panic attack by approximately 1-2 min, and became more intense while he was in a panic state. The patient strongly believed that he 'was going crazy,' but he did not proceed into any delusional elaboration of the hallucinations." The hallucinations lasted for about fifteen minutes. Within an hour, the ensuing panic attack had passed.

A team of Australian researchers looked more specifically at the link between auditory hallucinations and caffeine. In an experiment that studied the combination of stress and caffeine in a group with no psychiatric problems, the researchers' methods sound, perhaps, a bit stressful, depending on your tolerance for Christmas carols.

The subjects were divided into four groups: low caffeine/low stress, low caffeine/high stress, high caffeine/low stress, and high caffeine/ high stress. Stress levels were determined by a standardized perceived stress questionnaire, and the threshold for high caffeine use was set at more than two hundred milligrams per day (nearly three SCADs).

Subjects had to listen to Bing Crosby singing "White Christmas." Then they were told that the song, or a fragment of the song, might be embedded into a white-noise sample. They listened to white noise through headphones, and the researchers noted how many times the subjects heard the music. The catch is that the researchers never played "White Christmas" under the white noise. The high stress/ high caffeine group reported the most "false alarms"; they thought they heard the song even though it was not playing.

In their 2011 paper, the authors wrote, "The results demonstrated that high caffeine levels in association with high levels of stressful life events interacted to produce higher levels of 'hallucination' in non-clinical participants, indicating that further caution needs to be advised with the use of this overtly 'safe' drug."

Caffeine-induced hallucinations are mercifully rare. But researchers hope such accounts will help them understand the drug's actions at lower levels within the normal range for most Americans.

Beyond panic and hallucination, caffeine is, very rarely, associated with more extreme mental states. One case is recounted by Dr. Dawson Hedges, of Brigham Young University. In the journal *CNS Spectrums* in 2009, he wrote, "A 47-year old successful male farmer with no history of psychiatric hospitalization presented with a 7-year history of depression, diminished sleep to as little as 4 hours/night, poor energy, explosive anger, decreased concentration, decreased appetite, anhedonia [inability to experience pleasure], and feeling of worthlessness."

The farmer drank coffee, and plenty of it. Seven years before the doctor saw him he had increased his coffee intake from twelve cups to thirty-six cups daily. When Hedges first saw him, the patient was drinking a gallon of coffee every day. "There was no history of psychosis before the increase in coffee consumption, but after the increased consumption, the patient developed paranoia," Hedges wrote. The farmer felt that people were plotting to drive him away and steal his farm.

The farmer was also taking several antianxiety drugs: paroxetine, alprazolam, clonazepam, and propanol. And he had poor hygiene. But after tapering off coffee, he was a different man altogether. "Notably, the patient's psychosis resolved upon lowering caffeine intake, and no other features of schizophrenia or any other psychosis were present, sparing the patient from the potential adverse effects and cost of antipsychotic medication," the author wrote. Hedges recommended that medical professionals consider caffeinism as a possible cause in patients with chronic psychosis.

In the most extreme cases, people have blamed caffeine for violent impulses. In Kentucky, Woody Will Smith killed his wife in 2009 by strangling her with an extension cord. He believed she was having an affair, and he used caffeine to stay awake so she could not sneak away with their children. He blamed the murder on sleep deprivation and caffeine intoxication. The jury did not buy it.

The caffeine-intoxication defense worked better for Dan Noble. The Idaho man went to a Starbucks store on a December morning in 2009 and bought two of his usual sixteen-ounce coffee drinks (on credit—he had no wallet and was clad in pajamas and flip flops). Then, he drove to nearby Pullman, Washington, in his gold Trans Am. Driving erratically, he hit one pedestrian in a crosswalk, then hit another a block later. Each of the victims suffered a broken leg from the collision. When the police arrived, they were forced to Taser Noble to subdue him.

Noble was acquitted on all charges, including vehicular assault. The reason? Insanity, caffeine induced. Noble's attorney said he had a "rare bipolar disorder, with caffeine as the final trigger." A condition of his acquittal: no more coffee.

And then there was Kenneth Sands, a Washington man who groped a woman and three teenage girls at a volleyball game in October 2011. He blamed his actions on caffeine-induced psychosis, but it did not get him off the hook. He landed a five-month jail sentence.

Some of these examples are quirky, and the acute caffeine-related psychological problems are rare. But the take-home message here is that caffeine can really mess with your head.

CHAPTER 13

Therapeutic Doses

On October 10, 1859, Dr. Henry Fraser Campbell was called to a hotel in his hometown of Augusta, Georgia. There he found "Mr. F.H.T.," a twenty-four-year-old male, lying on a sofa in a clerk's office with his head resting in a friend's lap. The patient had taken an overdose of laudanum (a tincture of opium that was often used as an analgesic until the twentieth century), in "a fit of temporary depression."

Mr. F.H.T. was unresponsive. Campbell poured ice water on his head, pumped his stomach, and tried to keep him breathing. But the patient was failing. His breaths slowed to four per minute; his skin was purplish and cold. His muscles were so relaxed that his head rolled around on his neck and his tongue hung out of his mouth.

Finally, Campbell thought of using a stimulant. This is how he described it:

> *Strong Coffee* naturally presented itself to our mind, but the only infusion we could obtain at that time, was a rather weak infusion left from the supper at the hotel. It was clearly impossible for the patient to *swallow* anything, and we did not think it advisable to run the risk of introducing

the stomach tube in his present condition; we therefore
called for a syringe, but the weakness of the coffee caused
us to hesitate about using it, when, fortunately, the idea of
Caffeine occurred to us, and we sent immediately for that
preparation. . . . A small quantity of the Caffeine was
rubbed upon the tongue and to the inner surface of each
cheek. The patient was then laid upon his side, *and an injection of the coffee with a large quantity (afterwards ascer-
tained to be* TWENTY GRAINS) *of the Caffeine dissolved in
it, was administered by the rectum,* with a common syringe.

Twenty grains is a heavy dose of caffeine, about thirteen hundred
milligrams, or seventeen SCADs. Within an hour, Campbell said, the
patient was quite responsive indeed: "He was in the exercise of the
most active muscularity; pulling away from his attendants, pushing
them from his bed-side, jumping out of bed, and performing every
variety of movements in the most energetic and well co-ordinated
manner." Campbell was certain that the drug had caused the recovery,
attributing it to caffeine's effects on the muscular system. Although
people could not yet order it off the Internet, as we can today, caffeine
powder was already available in 1860 in Augusta, Georgia. And doctors were well aware of its stimulating effects.

⚡

Campbell's case was an early and graphic example of caffeine's
therapeutic uses beyond staying alert and running fast. Luckily, rectal
caffeine infusions are now as rare as depressed laudanum victims
languishing in the hotels of northeast Georgia. Although caffeine is
no longer prescribed for opiate overdoses, it does have therapeutic
applications, some surprising, some well-known.

Pediatricians often use caffeine to treat apnea (the cessation or in-
terruption of breathing) in premature infants. One study found that
premature infants treated with caffeine developed fewer cases of bron-

chopulmonary dysplasia, a serious lung disorder that is a common complication for premature babies. (Theophylline, the closely related chemical that is essentially unmethylated caffeine, can also be used to treat apnea, but it is less effective.)

The most common, and well-known, therapeutic application of caffeine is for relieving headaches. The drug's effects on headaches are complex, particularly since in some people caffeine actually triggers them. At least some of the ameliorating effect is due to its work as a vasoconstrictor—it contracts the blood vessels in the brain, thereby reducing the throbbing headache sensation.

Of course, a headache is often a symptom of caffeine withdrawal. Doctors have figured out that the headaches that so often plague hospitalized postoperative patients are often caused by caffeine withdrawal, due to imposed dietary restrictions. The good news is that the headaches are quickly alleviated with a caffeinated beverage.

Migraine sufferers can get relief from prescription medications like Fioricet, which bundles caffeine with acetaminophen and a barbiturate. Caffeine is so effective in treating migraine headaches that it's even bundled into a prescription suppository called Cafergot, for people too nauseated to hold down a pill. (Over-the-counter caffeine suppositories are also used by some Orthodox Jews, to alleviate withdrawal while fasting on Yom Kippur.) But one large study showed that even a nonprescription formula combining caffeine, aspirin, and acetaminophen was very effective in treating migraine headaches and associated symptoms.

Caffeine is more commonly used in popular over-the-counter analgesics like Excedrin and Anacin. The basic Anacin formula boasts "Aspirin + Caffeine = Fast Pain Relief." It incorporates 32 milligrams of caffeine per tablet, with two tablets as the recommended adult dose (nearly one SCAD). Excedrin Extra Strength caplets incorporate aspirin, acetaminophen, and caffeine (130 milligrams, nearly two SCADS, per recommended adult dose).

These pills are often considered fantastic hangover remedies. Anacin capitalizes on this with its trademarked slogan: "Great night. Rough morning. Better day." For younger hangover sufferers, there are energy drinks like Monster Rehab and Rockstar Recovery, delivering a bit of morning-after caffeine. And Hangover Joe's energy shots take the basic energy shot formula and package it for people who drank too much. Though it is padded with a lot of other ingredients (niacin, kudzu, etc.), its primary ingredient is caffeine, three SCADs' worth.

Other popular over-the-counter caffeine pills, like Dexatrim, promise to help dieters lose weight. These diet pills are often pushed by flavor-of-the-month celebrities: Kim Kardashian hawks QuickTrim, while Snooki is pushing Zantrex3. The trouble is, caffeine won't help you lose weight.

It is hard to understand why the pills include caffeine as the main ingredient, unless it is because caffeine is a stimulant, and people tend to associate stimulants with suppressing appetites. Terry Graham, the University of Guelph physiologist, said it may partly be due to a lingering belief that caffeine will help burn fat.

"It is such a popular myth," he said. Caffeine has even found its way into products like panty hose that promise, again falsely, to help slim your legs. "That's painless," Graham told me with a chuckle. "You'd better get them off before you disappear. I guess that's the only risk."

⚡

Beyond caffeine's medical applications, science keeps revealing more about how it affects our bodies and minds. Invariably, each new finding makes its way onto the science and health pages in newspapers, giving caffeine lovers reason to rejoice or despair, depending on the discovery of the day. But we don't need to be whipsawed by the findings, alternately reassured and freaked out; we just need to understand that caffeine is a complicated drug that can affect us in strange ways.

One pleasant surprise for coffee drinkers is that caffeine might ward off depression. For a study published in 2011 in *Archives of Inter-*

nal Medicine, Harvard researcher Dr. Alberto Ascherio and his colleagues mined data from the Nurses' Health Study to see if the consumption of caffeinated beverages is associated with the risk of depression. They only looked at women, who suffer depression twice as frequently as men (one in five will experience depression at some point in their lives).

Their analysis not only found that coffee drinkers suffered less from depression; it showed that those who drank the most coffee (more than four cups a day) suffered the least. "In this large prospective cohort of older women free of clinical depression or severe depressive symptoms at baseline, risk of depression decreased in a dose-dependent manner with increasing consumption of caffeinated coffee," they wrote. "Consumption of decaffeinated coffee was not associated with reduced risk of depression."

The authors did note a major limitation of the study. The subjects were first interviewed at a mean age of sixty-three, and then ten years later. Many of the people who develop depression would have done so by this age, and would have been excluded from the study. Too, it may be that depressive people have less of an appetite for coffee. So it is not possible to determine cause and effect. Still, the findings were enough to prompt this enthusiastic editor's note from Dr. Seth Berkowitz:

> This study makes an important contribution because it is, to my knowledge, the first large-scale study of coffee consumption to evaluate a mental health outcome in women. Previous work has focused mainly on the effects of caffeine on cardiovascular disease (generally finding no overall effect on cardiovascular disease incidence of mortality), inflammation (generally showing modest increases in markers of systemic inflammation), and particular types of malignant neoplasms, including breast cancer (generally showing no or modest protective effects). Taken together, these results reassure coffee drinkers that there

seem to exist no glaringly deleterious health consequences
to coffee consumption.

It is a definitive conclusion—given what we know now, coffee won't
kill you. But other recent studies suggest how much more we have to
learn. Strangely, another paper that looked at the association between
depression and coffee drinking, this time in men, came to a different
conclusion, suggesting that coffee, not caffeine, might be preventing
depression. The researchers found that "coffee consumption may reduce the risk for severe depression, whereas no association was found
for tea and caffeine intake."

In 2013, Dr. Ascherio and his Harvard colleagues published a paper
showing that drinking caffeinated coffee was associated with a reduced
risk of suicide. As with their study on depression in women, the risk
decreased as coffee consumption increased, with lowest suicide risk
among those who drank four or more cups daily (they assumed 137
milligrams of caffeine per eight-ounce cup of coffee, nearly two SCADs).
Again, they did not find the same association with decaf coffee.

A 2012 study suggested coffee drinking is linked to longer life. This
one, as you might imagine, got a lot of media attention. Researchers
with the National Cancer Institute at the National Institutes of Health
mined data on more than four hundred thousand Americans between
the ages of fifty and seventy-one. They found an association between
coffee drinking and a lower risk of death. Drinking three or more cups
of coffee was associated with a 10 percent lower risk of death.

But it is worth noting several things here. First of all, the study
only showed an association, not a cause-and-effect relationship. Second, decaffeinated coffee was actually more strongly associated with
decreased mortality than regular coffee, but both were significantly
better than no coffee. Finally, the authors did not distinguish among
the different types of brewing. The take-home message, in the words
of the authors: "Our results provide reassurance with respect to the
concern that coffee drinking might adversely affect health."

Researchers have also found a strong association between habitual coffee drinking and a substantially lower risk of type 2 diabetes. But caffeine is probably not the protective mechanism.

Just as the research on coffee and type 2 diabetes was being published, Terry Graham was seeing something that looked quite different. His research showed that caffeine promotes insulin resistance. Insulin is the hormone best known for its role in regulating blood sugar. Graham's studies showed that subjects' blood sugar levels were elevated after taking caffeine and carbohydrates.

He told me it was hard to reconcile his work showing that caffeine promotes insulin resistance with the studies showing that coffee is associated with a lower risk of type 2 diabetes.

"When this first started to come out, we were already publishing our work, and I was completely confused," he said. "As any objective scientist, I concluded the other guy was wrong and I was right. But in fact, that wasn't the case; we were both right."

He said there is no doubt about his findings: "Regardless of a person's caffeine or coffee habits, if we give an individual either caffeinated coffee or pure caffeine, and then a food or beverage that has carbohydrate in it, and they sit at rest, then, for a prolonged period of time—and I can't say how long, but certainly for a number of hours afterward—the individual becomes insulin resistant."

For healthy people, Graham said the insulin resistance is within the margin of safety. "I think of myself as a healthy, active person, and I drink coffee all the time and I never am concerned with, 'Oh, gee, there I've really insulted my body,' because I am quite confident that my body can produce that little bit of extra insulin and get the job done," he said. "But if I was a sedentary individual, if I was obese, if I had a family history for type 2 diabetes, or knew that I was moving in that direction, I would certainly be avoiding caffeine."

Conversely, this effect could be beneficial to type 1 diabetics when they experience the acute hypoglycemia known as insulin shock. Graham said a caffeinated soft drink would help raise blood sugar levels more than a non-caffeinated soft drink, which would be exactly what a hypoglycemic person would need at the time. Caffeine's relationship to insulin is another indication that the drug has many and varied effects throughout the body. Some are significant, others subtle, and greater awareness could really pay off in some cases.

In another surprising finding, Harvard researchers in 2012 found an association between the consumption of caffeinated coffee and a lower incidence of basal cell carcinoma, a type of skin cancer that is so common its rate of occurrence may soon equal the rate of occurrence of all other cancers combined. The lower incidence was associated with caffeinated coffee, not decaf, suggesting caffeine is the protective agent. While the effect was small, the doctors noted, "Given the nearly one million new cases diagnosed each year in the United States, modification in daily dietary factors with even small protective effects may have great public health impact." The exact protective mechanism is unclear, but mouse studies have shown that caffeine can help to eliminate sun-damaged skin cells.

Perhaps the biggest worry about caffeine has been that it might cause birth defects or miscarriages. In the late 1980s, these were some of the concerns that prompted a federally appointed committee to suggest reevaluating its use in soft drinks. And the studies have piled up continually ever since.

In an effort to make sense of the studies, the American College of Obstetricians and Gynecologists' Committee on Obstetric Practice issued a committee opinion in 2010. Their conclusion: "Moderate caffeine consumption (less than 200 mg per day) does not appear to be a major contributing factor in miscarriage or pre-term birth. The relationship of caffeine to growth restriction remains undetermined. A final conclusion cannot be made at this time as to whether there is a correlation between high caffeine intake and miscarriage."

But any aspiring mothers who were placated by the opinion, and comforted by the news that they do not have to forego caffeine entirely, got unwelcome news in early 2013 when a team of Scandinavian researchers published a paper stating that "caffeine intake was consistently associated with decreased BW [birth weight] and increased odds of SGA [the baby being small for gestational age]." And it was not just the higher doses that had an effect. The authors found that caffeine consumption of less than two hundred milligrams per day was associated with a higher risk of a baby being born small.

It is worth noting that this study does not actually contradict the conclusion of the obstetricians' committee, who found that the "relationship of caffeine to growth restriction remains undetermined."

Another caffeine quirk that is of more interest to women: In 2012, researchers found that moderate caffeine consumption is associated with changes in estrogen levels, but in different ways. White women who consumed two hundred milligrams of caffeine or more daily had lower levels of estrogen than their non-caffeinated counterparts; Asian women showed the opposite trend. But strangely, different sources of caffeine affected estrogen levels differently. Among those who took less caffeine, from sources other than coffee, a daily serving of green tea or caffeinated soda was associated with higher estrogen levels among Asians, blacks, and whites. (In all cases, the changes were not sufficient to affect ovulation.)

For years scientists believed that caffeine could contribute to osteoporosis, the loss of bone density in older people, which disproportionately affects women. Caffeine does slightly depress the stomach's ability to absorb calcium, and some doctors had worried that the drug could contribute to reduced bone mass and increased fracture risk. But this is not the case, according to endocrinologist Robert Heaney. "The negative effect of caffeine on calcium absorption is small enough to be fully offset by as little as 1–2 tablespoons of milk," he wrote in a 2002 paper. "All of the observations implicating caffeine-containing beverages as a risk factor for osteoporosis have been made in populations consuming substantially less than optimal calcium intakes."

And here is more news that older coffee drinkers, or coffee drinkers who hope to grow older, should appreciate: Research suggests that caffeine might play a role in staving off Parkinson's and Alzheimer's diseases. A 2000 study analyzing data from eight thousand Japanese-American men found a lower incidence of Parkinson's disease among coffee drinkers. And here it seemed to be the caffeine that did the trick. The scientists wrote, "The data suggest that the mechanism is related to caffeine intake and not to other nutrients contained in coffee."

In 2010, a team of researchers from Portugal and Spain reviewed the available studies on Alzheimer's and caffeine. Their findings were nuanced. Although they found a trend toward a protective effect of caffeine, the researchers said the studies were so varied that they precluded "robust and definite statements on this topic."

In both cases, the data cannot show that caffeine caused the lower incidence of disease. It could be that the neurology of people who are vulnerable to these neurodegenerative disorders makes them less inclined to consume caffeine. And if caffeine is conferring a neuroprotective effect, it is not yet clear exactly which of its mechanisms might be responsible. Researchers suspect it is related to caffeine's influence on adenosine and dopamine.

Scientists are constantly learning, and even seeing, more about how caffeine swamps adenosine receptors. In 2012, David Elmenhorst and his colleagues in Germany used neuroimaging to understand just how many of the primary adenosine receptors are plugged up with caffeine in conditions of normal use. They studied A1 receptors, which are the most widespread adenosine receptors in the human brain and are abundant in the cortex. Cortical neurons are important for higher cognitive function. The A2A receptors, which are associated with the genetic variant that gives some people panic attacks, are more confined to areas deeper in the brain, in the basal ganglia.

"There is still an ongoing debate about which of these receptors is more relevant for the action of caffeine," Elmenhorst told me. "Some studies are hinting for the A1, and some are more for the A2A."

The researchers administered caffeine intravenously to fifteen male subjects, at concentrations raging from one milligram per kilogram to four milligrams per kilogram of body mass (for a 150-pound person, that is a range of about one to four SCADs). The paper includes some very cool images of the brain with and without caffeine, showing how the drug saturates neuroreceptors. Elmenhorst said his was the first human study to show that the doses of caffeine we commonly consume block about 50 percent of our adenosine receptors.

Fifty percent is actually an important figure, emphasized Elmenhorst. When you are looking for drugs to treat psychiatric disorders like, say, schizophrenia, you want something that will occupy about 60 to 70 percent of the targeted receptors. That is usually a level high enough to give you a therapeutic dose, but below the threshold that leads to unpleasant side effects. It is another indication that the habitual use of coffee, tea, cola, or energy drinks can be seen as self-administration of the drug. "I think people are intuitively dosing themselves with the right dose of caffeine that has good actions and low side effects," Elmenhorst told me.

We've seen that individual differences affect the way we each metabolize caffeine. Birth control pills, smoking, and genetic predispositions in genes governing adenosine processing and enzyme production are some of the factors. Another is personality type. More specifically, the traits of introversion and extroversion, originally described by the Swiss psychiatrist Carl Jung. Extroverts are seen as sociable, assertive, and gregarious. Introverts have more of an inward focus and often prefer solitary activities. It has long been understood that extroverts get more cognitive enhancement from caffeine. For a study published in 2013, researchers assessed subjects' abilities to recall letters they had seen earlier and react by pressing the appropriate button on a keyboard. They found that caffeine enhanced working memory for extroverts, but it did not help introverts' performance.

Another oddity about caffeine is the way that knowing you are consuming it can increase its effect. Why is this? It has to do with what psychologists call "expectancy." To test this effect, Lynne Dawkins led a team of British researchers that divided eighty-eight subjects into four groups and gave them coffee. One group was given caffeinated coffee and was told it was caffeinated. The second group got caffeinated coffee and was told it was decaf. The third group got decaf and was told it was caffeinated. The last group got decaf and knew it was decaf. In all cases, the caffeinated brew had approximately seventy-five milligrams of caffeine (one SCAD) per serving.

In this way, the researchers were testing coffee's placebo effect: a measurable improvement based solely on the perception that a treatment will be beneficial. (This is the effect that double-blind studies protect against, because both the subject and the researcher are unaware of the actual contents of the administered dose.) Earlier studies had found that expectancy improved sustained attention only when caffeine was actually consumed—a synergistic effect of the caffeine plus the expectancy of consuming it. Dawkins's team found otherwise; she wrote, "The present findings did not support this view; we found performance enhancement by expectation of coffee regardless of whether caffeinated or decaffeinated coffee had been consumed."

Indeed, on one test, expectation eclipsed caffeine. The Stroop effect is a phenomenon in which we more quickly read the word *red*, for example, if it is printed in red ink (when it is known as "congruent") than if it is printed in blue ink ("incongruent"). The Stroop test measures cognitive function by recording how many correct responses you have when asked to identify both types of words, often in a specified amount of time.

"Overall, the findings from the Stroop task suggest that expectation of having consumed caffeine confers an enhancement of sustained attention that is at least comparable, and perhaps superior to, pharmacological effects of caffeine," Dawkins wrote.

OK, so these findings are of limited practical use. Unless, of course, you want to cut down on caffeine and you can find someone to serve you decaf and tell you it is caffeinated coffee. In that case, you would likely do better work than if you knew you were drinking decaf. But the work goes a long way toward understanding why we want that cup of coffee in our hand at crunch time. As Dawkins wrote, "Both caffeine and expectation of having consumed caffeine improved attention and psychomotor speed. Expectation enhanced self-reported vigour and reward responsivity."

But caffeine has still more surprises for us. Let's say you are an extrovert, your adenosine receptors are optimally swamped with caffeine, and you've got a cup of coffee in hand, to boot, so you are feeling just right. Meeting with a coworker to discuss a project, you are firing on all cylinders. Then something reminds you of an old college friend. You can picture him but you can't remember his name. You might be able to blame the caffeine.

This frustrating experience of knowing an answer but being temporarily unable to recall it is known to cognitive scientists as the "tip-of-tongue effect." While caffeine enhances recall for words related to the immediate train of thought, which is not really surprising, it actually increases the tip-of-tongue effect for unrelated words.

Researchers Valerie Lesk and Stephen Womble, of Trieste, Italy, tested the recall of thirty-two college students with or without two hundred milligrams of caffeine. Tested on one hundred general-knowledge questions, the students with caffeine had fewer tip-of-tongue experiences than the control group, but only for words related to a target group. Trying to name unrelated words gave them the inverse effect—more of those frustrating tip-of-tongue responses.

It is these complicated and highly varied effects that make caffeine so hard to pigeonhole. And they go a long way toward explaining why, for more than a century, American regulators have simply not known what to do with caffeine.

PART IV

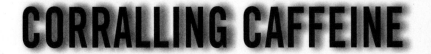

CORRALLING CAFFEINE

CHAPTER 14

Unleashing the Beasts

For more than sixty years, from the resolution of the Chattanooga trial until the late 1970s, regulators pretty much left caffeine alone. Meanwhile, the soft drink industry exploded while coffee consumption peaked and fell.

In 1958, the FDA adopted the Food Additives Amendment to the Federal Food, Drug, and Cosmetic Act, which formally granted caffeine GRAS status. That is the FDA acronym for "generally recognized as safe," meaning the additive had a long history of safe use in food. But the FDA said caffeine was GRAS only for "cola-type beverages" and only at concentrations below 0.02 percent, or 200 parts per million. That is the equivalent of 71 milligrams per 12-ounce serving, or roughly double the concentration in a modern can of Coke (although the pre-Chattanooga Coca-Cola would have exceeded this threshold). In a 1966 regulation defining "soda water," the FDA actually made caffeine a mandatory ingredient of some soft drinks. The standard required that soda water, "which includes the word 'cola' or a designation as a 'pepper' beverage that, for years, has become well known as being made with kola nut extract and thus as a caffeine-containing drink, shall contain caffeine in a quantity not to exceed 0.02 percent by weight."

Caffeine ran into trouble in 1978, when a federal committee tasked with reviewing its safety suggested the GRAS status be revoked. To reduce speculation about caffeine's effects, the committee called for "a series of rigorously controlled chronic studies in appropriate species, including fetal, neonatal, and growing animals, of the immediate and ultimate behavioral and cardiovascular effects of caffeine added to the diet and given in cola-type beverages." The committee did not look into coffee and tea; it was only concerned with caffeine's safety as a food additive.

In 1980, taking up the committee's suggestion, the FDA proposed stripping caffeine of its GRAS status and suggested a series of studies on animals and humans to better understand the health risks. The FDA's reconsideration of caffeine opened up a can of worms. Coca-Cola got nervous. Pepsi got nervous. Even the National Coffee Association got sucked in.

In a letter to the FDA, NCA's president George E. Boecklin wrote, "While the proposed regulation does not cover coffee, the underlying scientific issues raised by the proposal are relevant to the safety of caffeine in food generally. The National Coffee Association therefore, has a significant interest in the correct resolution of these issues."

When Coca-Cola responded to the FDA, it based its opposition on the company's long-standing use of the same formula. It appended a 1958 letter that FDA deputy commissioner John Harvey had written to Coca-Cola senior vice president Edgar Forio, to reassure him that the then-pending Food Additives Amendment would not affect it. Harvey had written, "The beverage Coca-Cola has been, in our opinion, in such common use for such a long period of time that its safety, as well as the safety of its components, is well-established by this history of food experience."

Ultimately, the proposal went nowhere. After scientific review assuaged most of the concerns about caffeine's carcinogenic and reproductive effects, the FDA let it languish for two decades and eventually dropped it in 2004. It died with a whimper, expunged as part of a routine culling of moribund regulatory efforts. Caffeine stayed on the GRAS list.

Along the way, something strange happened. The FDA had recognized that many soft drinks did not fit the cola definition in its soda water regulations. Some, like Mountain Dew, were caffeinated but not flavored with kola nut; others, like caffeine-free Coke, were cola flavored but had no caffeine. After first trying to rewrite the definition of cola-type beverages, the FDA decided in 1989 to simply nix the standard of identity for soda water that included cola-type beverages. That left the GRAS standard for caffeine with a significant gap, which remains today—it references cola-type beverages, but the FDA has no regulatory standard defining such a drink.

The controversy did contribute to greater caffeine awareness in the early 1980s. Sales of decaffeinated coffee spiked. This was the era when Maxwell House invested millions to build the Houston decaffeination tower now run by Maximus. The decaf brand Brim ran TV ads that said, "Fill your cup with flavor, not caffeine." Sanka, the decaf pioneer whose name derived from the French *sans caféine*, was huge in the 1980s. It took a comedic star turn in the film *Fast Times at Ridgemont High*, when a beleaguered science teacher implored his students, "Look, I'm a little slow today. I just switched to Sanka, so have a heart." The brand developed TV ads showing an uptight man whose wife has to explain, "His doctor says that caffeine makes him tense." Brim ran similar ads, with the message, "My doctor says caffeine makes me nervous."

A series of ads for 7UP featuring the Trinidadian actor Geoffrey Holder saying, "7UP is light and refreshing. Crisp and clean, and no caffeine. Never had it, never will." It also used the slogan "You don't need caffeine, and neither does your cola." (The Seven-Up Company wound up in court when RC Cola bottlers Royal Crown Cola Company asserted the anti-caffeine claims jeopardized its reputation.) Coca-Cola ran newspaper ads showing cans of caffeine-free Coke, Diet Coke, and Tab reading, "Now, caffeine-free drinks that taste like they aren't caffeine-free."

The controversy spawned the International Life Sciences Institute, a nonprofit formed with industry support for the purpose of studying caffeine. The ILSI has grown into a large, industry-funded nonprofit, with a broad and honorable mission: "to improve public health and well being." Its various committees are staffed by the world's largest food and beverage conglomerates. The caffeine committee includes representatives from Coca-Cola, Pepsi, Red Bull, Kraft, Mars, and Unilever.

The tussle also generated thousands of pages of correspondence between the FDA and the soft drink companies, and their lawyers and scientists, including such arcana as a paper titled "Caffeine Does Not Bind Covalently to Liver Microsomes from Different Animal Species and to Proteins and DNA from Perfused Rat Liver."

Many dozens of the pages in the FDA's files came from an advocate for healthy foods, who has been a thorn in the sides of soft drink companies for decades.

Michael Jacobson, the director of the Center for Science in the Public Interest, is a crusader in the mold of Harvey Wiley. He swings for the fences, makes powerful corporate enemies who delight in ridiculing his claims, and is not prone to compromise. It was Jacobson who alerted Americans to the heart-clogging properties of movie popcorn in 1994, when he stated that a large serving had as much saturated fat as six Big Macs.

Jacobson has been trying to get Americans to eat better since the early 1970s, when he and two other newly minted PhDs met through their work with Ralph Nader. "We thought it would be interesting to start an organization that was run by scientists, both to emphasize the science and also to inspire other scientists to get involved in social issues," Jacobson told me. "Of course, we didn't know anything about starting an organization or getting funding, so we're pretty lucky to have survived." The center has done more than survive—by 2012 it boasted sixty full-time employees in a large suite of offices on L Street, near the Capitol in Washington, D.C., and an annual budget of $17 million.

Slight and bespectacled, with a curly gray mane, Jacobson speaks gently but has a way with words. He coined the term "liquid candy" to describe soft drinks. Some people even credit him with coining the term "junk food," although he says that isn't so. "Thinking back to the early 1970s, what distinguished us from most of the other people who were talking about food safety and nutrition was that they spoke in euphemisms and academic terms. We would talk about Coke and Pepsi, rather than 'carbonated soft drinks,' because brand names resonate with people; generic terms don't."

His campaigns against salt, fat, and sugar have made Jacobson an easy target for opponents of regulations—the Center for Consumer Freedom calls him "nanny in chief"—but he remains unfazed. "The criticisms of us—'All you want is a nanny state' and 'Don't take my Coke away from me'—typically it's from industry and industry's allies," said Jacobson. "At some point, the government and companies have to acknowledge the science: that trans fat is killing us. That salt is killing us. That we have an obesity epidemic."

Way back in the late 1970s, when Starbucks had just a few Seattle cafés and nobody had heard of energy drinks, Jacobson already perceived an emerging caffeine problem. In 1979, shortly after the select committee raised concerns about caffeine, Jacobson petitioned the FDA to tighten caffeine regulations.

His July 1981 comments to the FDA about the GRAS status of caffeine included a passage that now seems prescient (remember, this was more than thirty years ago, when Ronald Reagan was starting his first term as president and the big news was the wedding of Prince Charles and Lady Diana). Jacobson wrote, "In the past fifteen years, caffeine has appeared in an increasing variety of soft drinks. In addition to cola and pepper beverages, orange- (Sunkist) and apple-flavored (Aspen) sodas contain caffeine, as do Mountain Dew and Mello Yello.

Manufacturers are clamoring to use caffeine. . . . In the next ten years, while the safety of caffeine is being questioned, more and more beverages consumed by children will contain caffeine."

In 1983, that Coca-Cola ad touting caffeine-free soft drinks prompted Jacobson to send another letter to the FDA. "For years, the soft drink industry, led by the Coca-Cola Company, has urged that caffeine . . . is necessary to provide the customary and desired flavor," he wrote. Then, ever so gently tweaking the beverage giant, he continued, "The FDA has been in the middle of the caffeine/soda pop controversy: Should flavor considerations outweigh health risks to children? We are pleased to report that good old American ingenuity has solved this problem. The Coca-Cola Company has announced that it can produce 'Caffeine free drinks that taste like they aren't caffeine free.' . . . Now that Coca-Cola has made this great breakthrough in flavor chemistry, we urge FDA to ban the addition of caffeine to soda pop to protect children's health." (This controversy over the importance of flavor also provided the impetus for Roland Griffiths's 2000 paper on the topic, described in chapter 5.)

It took the FDA sixteen years to deny Jacobson's first caffeine petition. He promptly filed another in 1997. In his second petition to the FDA, Jacobson listed some of caffeine's ills—including sleeplessness, anxiety, and addiction—to make the case for better labeling. More specifically, he asked the FDA to require that foods and beverages not only list caffeine as an ingredient but also divulge the quantity.

During this time, there was some gentlemanly unpleasantness between Jacobson and the FDA. Responding to a 1980 missive about the proposed GRAS revision, FDA acting director Dr. Mark Novitch wrote Jacobson, saying he shared some of Jacobson's concerns about caffeine. He wrote, "FDA has carefully evaluated all the available evidence and has concluded that a warning label on coffee and tea is not justified at this time. Although you have apparently reached a different judgment on this issue, I cannot accept your characterization of FDA's position as 'irresponsible.'"

But any enmity has mostly been smoothed over. In 1996, FDA commissioner David Kessler (the one who brought the issue of nicotine to a head) even awarded Jacobson the agency's Special Citation, which read, "Presented to Michael F. Jacobson for helping government, industry, and the public understand the relationship between diet and health and, in doing so, accomplishing one of the great public health advances of the century." The accompanying bronze medal bore the likeness of the first forceful anti-caffeine advocate in America: Harvey Wiley.

The FDA has yet to act on Jacobson's second petition. But after thirty years of advocacy, he did finally score a caffeine coup. In 2008, he filed suit against Anheuser-Busch and Miller Brewing Company for marketing alcoholic drinks with added caffeine. Jacobson claimed Miller marketed Sparks drinks as "high-fun" beverages with an "irreverent tone." Anheuser-Busch was also in the game, with Tilt and Bud Extra. Jacobson called the products "alcospeed." Also under pressure by a group of attorneys general, the bottlers ultimately settled with Jacobson's organization and the state attorneys, and pulled the products from the market. But Sparks and Tilt never got enough traction in the marketplace to generate much negative press for caffeinated alcohol. That came soon enough, though, when the blends were popularized by dozens of smaller, independent bottlers, including one whose brand became rather infamous. This controversy marked the first time the FDA would flex its regulatory muscle over the new breeds of caffeinated products.

In the fall of 2010, nine Central Washington University students landed in an emergency room, nearly comatose after drinking a canned blend of caffeine and alcohol called Four Loko. More than a dozen others wound up in an ER in Lancaster, Pennsylvania. A twenty-one-year-old woman in Maryland died when she crashed her pickup after drinking two cans of the caffeinated alcohol. Bellevue Hospital Center,

in Manhattan, saw a slew of young men who had overindulged—one
had fallen onto subway tracks. Suddenly, it seemed, the nation was
awash in a new health threat, and the brew dubbed "blackout in a can"
grabbed headlines for weeks.

Each 24-ounce can of Four Loko contained 156 milligrams of caffeine (two SCADS) and as much alcohol as nearly five 12-ounce
beers. Fans said the caffeine and alcohol mixture allowed them to
party all night. Because of its stimulant effect, some called it "liquid
cocaine."

Four Loko was as inevitable as it was dangerous. When energy
drinks emerged in the 1990s, they soon became popular as cocktail
mixers. Drinks like Red Bull and vodka, and the Jagermeister and Red
Bull blends called "Jager Bombs," exploded in popularity. It was not
long before enterprising bottlers thought to sell the premixed blends
of caffeinated alcohol. After Jacobson and the attorneys general forced
Budweiser and Miller out of the market, smaller, independent companies like Four Loko bottler Phusion Projects began to flood it.

Dr. Mary Claire O'Brien was not surprised by the rash of emergency room visits—she had predicted it. Even before Four Loko became popular O'Brien had seen victims of caffeine-and-alcohol binges
in her emergency room in Winston-Salem, North Carolina. A curious
and observant doctor and associate professor of emergency medicine
at Wake Forest University, O'Brien quickly became one of the most
articulate critics of the drinks.

In a 2006 survey of more than four thousand students from ten
North Carolina universities conducted by O'Brien, nearly a quarter
said they mixed alcohol with energy drinks. O'Brien's survey showed
that the students who mixed alcohol and energy drinks were more
likely to engage in risky behaviors: being taken advantage of sexually,
taking advantage of another sexually, or riding with an alcohol-
impaired driver. They were also more likely to get injured or require
medical treatment. O'Brien said these behaviors might be rooted in
the fact that caffeinated drunks are less aware of their intoxication. In

addition, caffeine does nothing to counteract the impairment caused by alcohol, and its adenosine-blocking effect reduces the sense of fatigue in drinkers, allowing them to drink more without passing out and giving them more energy to do dangerous things. She said the research on mixing caffeine and alcohol suggests "a significant association between the consumption of those very heavily caffeinated products and serious alcohol-related injury. And clearly with drinking well in excess of what would otherwise be tolerated."

The Four Loko controversy triggered more caffeine research. In Gainesville, Bruce Goldberger—the forensic toxicologist who has long quantified caffeine levels in products ranging from Starbucks coffee to energy shots—enlisted a team to interview more than twelve hundred people leaving bars late at night. His findings were striking. He found that people who mixed caffeine and alcohol were three times as likely to leave the bar highly intoxicated and four times as likely to plan to drive a car after leaving the bar district. Goldberger's observations were troubling, but they only showed that the drinks were associated with risky behavior; he could not say that the combination of two popular drugs caused the behavior. (Another explanation could be that people who are more likely to drink to excess and drive are simply more attracted to energy drinks.)

The caffeinated alcohol also piqued Roland Griffiths's interest. He initiated a parametric study at Johns Hopkins, observing subjects' self-administration and performance while manipulating the doses of caffeine and alcohol in a lab setting.

In 2009, the year before the Four Loko controversy peaked with the flood of emergency room visits, O'Brien and other scientists, and seventeen attorneys general, had petitioned the FDA to ban these products. That prompted the agency to mail letters to twenty-seven bottlers in November 2009, saying caffeine had never been deemed generally recognized as safe (GRAS) for use in alcoholic beverages and the burden was on the manufacturers to prove that the products were safe according to scientific evidence and expert opinion. But still the drinks stayed on store shelves, and all those dozens of caffeine-amped inebriates landed in emergency rooms.

Finally, in November 2010, the FDA mailed out warning letters to the bottlers of Four Loko and other caffeinated alcohol blends. "It is FDA's view that the caffeine content of your beverages could result in central nervous system effects if a consumer drank one or more containers of your product," the letter read. "Therefore, FDA believes that the consumption of your products . . . may result in adverse behavioral outcomes because the caffeine is likely to counteract some, but not all, of the adverse effects of alcohol." The FDA claimed the right to seize the products and prosecute the bottlers. The cans came off the shelves.

Americans have a long history of mixing alcohol and caffeine. Long before Sparks and Four Loko, there was Kahlua, lightly caffeinated—approximately ten milligrams per serving—by dint of its coffee content. And then there is Allen's Coffee Flavored Brandy, the drink of choice for generations of Mainers. Allen's is not just the top-selling liquor in Maine; its various sizes occupy four of the top ten sales rungs. Mainers drink a million bottles annually, and statewide sales in 2011 exceeded $11 million.

The drink has inspired Facebook pages, tribute songs, and nicknames like "Rockland martini" and "gorilla juice." Bar patrons ask for "Allen's and milk," "a milk drink," "a brandy," or simply "an Allen's." Some call it a Sombrero, but it all means the same thing: equal parts coffee brandy and milk, on ice, in a pint glass. The most ominous moniker, "burnt trailer," refers to the mayhem that ensues when rural Mainers drink too much coffee brandy. (In a strange parallel, Buckfast Tonic Wine, a beloved Scottish drink with high levels of caffeine and alcohol, has earned the moniker "wreck the hoose juice.")

Some coffee brandy fans say the drink gives them energy to party all night. But Gary Shaw, a vice president at M. S. Walker, which bottles the brandy in Somerville, Massachusetts, told me that is a misconception. He said the drink contains some caffeine as a by-product of natural coffee flavoring, but could not say exactly how much.

Coffee brandy is more than a regional oddity. It illustrates some of the distinctions the Food and Drug Administration makes among caffeinated drinks: Add caffeinated coffee to a drink and it is considered a natural flavor; blend in some caffeine powder and it is another beast entirely. As we'll see, it's a distinction that is increasingly getting blurred.

Although the Four Loko case cracked open the regulatory door, the FDA did not see it as an opportunity to set meaningful caffeine standards for nonalcoholic products. The FDA did not claim alcoholic energy drink bottlers exceeded any regulatory caffeine limits; rather, that it does not consider caffeine to be GRAS when added to alcohol, at any concentration. The FDA's actions offered no new guidance on safe levels of caffeine in beverages, or whether the caffeine content should be better labeled.

Anyway, the FDA would soon have bigger fish to fry. Monsters, even.

When you crack a can of Monster Energy, you first hear the hiss of the escaping carbonation. Poured into a glass, Monster is about the color of a pale ale. On the tongue . . . well, it's an acquired taste: slightly metallic, syrupy sweet, a faint hint of orange Creamsicle. No, it's not a hot cup of Colombian, but you could get used to it. Millions of Americans have.

With a striking logo of three neon green claw marks and the slogan "unleash the beast," Monster energy drinks seem suddenly to be everywhere. In 2011, Monster surpassed Red Bull in energy drink sales in the United States, by volume, according to *Beverage Digest*. While the beverage industry tends to be masterful at marketing, few companies have done better than Monster.

Monster evolved from a product called Hansen's Energy, introduced by the California juice company Hansen's Naturals in 1997, the same year Red Bull launched its drinks in the United States. Initially, Red Bull clobbered its American competitor, but Hansen's soon clawed its way into the market. Sales started out slowly, but took off in 2002 when

Hansen's hired McLean Design, a Bay Area firm, to improve their marketing efforts—which they did in three specific ways, to great effect.

McLean came up with the Monster name, its memorable slogan, and the distinctive logo. (The claw-mark logo is now a very popular tattoo, even among high school students.) It also recommended the tried-and-true American marketing tradition of supersizing. Hansen's made its Monster cans twice the size of a Red Bull, but charged the same price. Then, they went to work promoting Monster with a marketing strategy like those of other energy drinks, targeting young males with an energetic blend of heavy metal bands, action-sports festivals, and bikini models.

Targeting young males for a caffeine-rich product makes sense, from a metabolic perspective. Jennifer Temple, of the University at Buffalo, studied gender differences in caffeine's reinforcement effects on adolescents. In a placebo-controlled double-blind study, males showed a stronger preference for caffeinated soda than did females. (Remember, reinforcement increases the likelihood that you will repeat a behavior.) "These data suggest that boys may be more susceptible to the reinforcing effects of caffeine," Temple wrote.

Whether or not it's got a metabolic basis, it's safe to say that Monster's marketing worked pretty well. Within seven years, it was a billion-dollar brand. By early 2012, Monster accounted for more than 90 percent of Hansen's sales, and the company acknowledged this by changing its name to Monster Beverage Corporation. The beast had swallowed the natural juice company. Monster had sales of nearly $2.4 billion in 2012.

Monster's effective slogan and logo jibed with a long tradition of companies trying to sell their caffeine delivery mechanisms in a crowded, saturated marketplace. Advertising and caffeine have long gone hand in glove. Sure we love our caffeine, but we are also constantly prodded with messages to love it a bit more. In fact, it is hard to find a corner store without prominent Coke or Pepsi logos, not just in the United States, but worldwide.

In Mexico, every roadhouse had stencils reading *"Toma lo bueno"* inside the iconic Coca-Cola bottle shape, or the Pepsi slogan *"Refresca tu mundo,"* with the *o* filled in with the tricolor Pepsi logo. In Shijiazhuang, China, the snack food kiosks were topped with huge Coke banners.

When I went to Maryland to talk to the FDA about caffeine regulations, I was greeted by a billboard for Sheets, the caffeinated gel strip company co-owned by NBA star LeBron James. On the east side of Baltimore, near Roland Griffiths's office, there was a big billboard with a McDonald's ad for a "breakfast sidekick"—$1 coffee, any size. And when I drove to Boston from the army research center in Natick, there were billboards advertising SK Energy, the shots developed by the rapper 50 Cent.

Understanding the scope and scale of the industry that is marketing caffeine may be the best way to see how culturally enmeshed it is and hints at the difficulties facing any regulators who set out to challenge it.

Ads for caffeine delivery mechanisms are everywhere you look—even in the *New York Times*. (In 2011, Starbucks swung a deal to be the only sponsor of the paper's digital home page for two days and bought so many full-page ads in the paper that it seemed more sponsor than advertiser.) 5-hour Energy has been underwriting NPR's *All Things Considered*, of all things.

Historically, the marketing has been a duel between cola and coffee, which was most pronounced in the early 1970s, before cola had passed coffee in per capita consumption. That's when the catchy "I'd like to buy the world a Coke" ad went head-to-head with Juan Valdez during episodes of *Columbo* or *The Partridge Family*. In the early 1980s, the National Coffee Association tried to reach out to a new generation of coffee drinkers with its Coffee Achievers TV ads, featuring David Bowie, Kurt Vonnegut, the rock band Heart, and the actress Cicely Tyson. But now the marketing is far more tightly targeted. Monster, for example, does not advertise in mass media, but has a remarkable presence online and gets its message out by promoting action sports events and sponsoring athletes.

The Portland, Oregon, advertising powerhouse Wieden and Kennedy, best known for coining the Nike catchphrase "Just do it," buttered its bread for years with the Coca-Cola and Starbucks accounts. It parted ways with the latter in 2008 over creative differences, but that contract illustrates where the juice is in the modern caffeine economy—the Starbucks account was worth $37 million in 2007; the Coca-Cola account was eleven times as valuable, worth $411 million.

Green Mountain Coffee Roasters spreads its ad money around in the Northeast. New York's Brand Buzz handles the coffee account and coined the clever phrase "a revelation in every cup," and Boston ad agency Brand Content has the Keurig account. In an effort to retain customers who might flee to Green Mountain, Starbucks, or other gourmet coffee brands, Folgers rolled out a massive TV, print, and Web campaign advertising its line of gourmet K-Cups with the help of Saatchi & Saatchi New York (the agency that long ago coined the jingle "The best part of waking up, is Folgers in your cup").

Dunkin' Donuts, aiming to increase the four million cups of coffee it serves daily, in 2011 assigned a multimillion-dollar ad campaign to the old-school Boston ad agency Hill Holliday. For its part, McDonald's in 2009 launched a $100 million campaign—its biggest ad blitz since rolling out breakfast sandwiches in the 1970s—to promote McCafés, its in-house coffee shops.

Caffeine is also getting plenty of product placement in movies. When Oliver Stone made *Wall Street: Money Never Sleeps*, Starbucks wanted its coffee featured in the film but came in too late; Dunkin' Donuts had already paid for the privilege. And the movie may have featured a silver screen first. In an awkward scene that looked like a bad commercial, an actor chugged a 5-hour Energy shot, the small label clearly visible. 5-hour Energy also has an aggressive print ad campaign, targeting seniors via full-page ads in AARP magazine. (On the other end of the age spectrum, Honey Boo Boo Child, a six-year-old breakout star of the TV show *Toddlers and Tiaras* who now has her own reality series, gets pumped up with a caffeinated drink mixture she calls "go-go juice.")

In 2007, Pepsi launched Pepsi Max in the United States with a marketing campaign by BBDO that *Advertising Age* estimated at $55 million. The campaign, which included Super Bowl ads, was clever but muddled. Pepsi Max began as a diet soda marketed to men, but soon dropped the "diet" from its name. It was unclear why the company had invested so much to launch a new cola in an already saturated market.

The first ad campaign gave a hint. The TV ads showed people nodding off uncomfortably, until they drank some Pepsi Max and began dancing around. The voice-over said, "Diet Pepsi Max, with ginseng and more caffeine." By creating a drink with caffeine levels higher than those of other colas but less than in energy drinks, Pepsi was hedging its bets against the threat of new FDA rules.

You'll recall that the FDA guideline for colas permits seventy-one milligrams of caffeine per twelve-ounce serving. Pepsi opted to blend sixty-nine milligrams into Pepsi Max (just as Jolt Cola had done twenty years before). If the FDA chooses to enforce its GRAS standard as a firm limit, Pepsi will have compliant products on the shelves, albeit at the maximum legal limit. Coca-Cola has tried the same strategy: Its Vault line also had caffeine levels just below the GRAS standard, but it failed to catch on and the company killed it.

The Diet Pepsi Max ads were atypical because they mentioned caffeine. Consistently and conspicuously absent from most ads for caffeinated products is any mention of the ingredient that gives them their appeal. You will never see much mention of it at Starbucks, for example. Starbucks CEO Howard Schultz's book *Onward* is full of stories about coffee's mystical allure, but it includes just one dismissive reference to caffeine. Some energy drink bottlers tend to blur the issue by talking about all the other ingredients in the beverages, like B vitamins, taurine, amino acids, and L-carnitine. The trouble is that none of these increase the energy drinks' kick.

Harris Lieberman and a colleague wrote this after reviewing the available literature on the subject: "At this time, there is little, if any, solid evidence to support an increase in either physical or mental 'energy' due to consumption of these drinks, except for the increases attributable to the caffeine in these products." The other ingredients, in other words, are window dressing, there to pad the labels, or to distract from the caffeine.

Downplaying caffeine's role is disingenuous, but entirely understandable. Caffeine is a drug, so to admit that a drug is the primary attraction in any product is fraught with both regulatory and moral peril. But there is another reason to divert the public's attention from caffeine's key role in commerce. If Starbucks acknowledged the caffeine's importance, then it would be more difficult to charge four dollars for a coffee drink. Consumers might prefer a Jet Alert tablet (you could buy a hundred for less than the price of a double latte). Starbucks Refreshers drinks, with fifty milligrams of caffeine, could easily be replaced at half price by a Diet Mountain Dew.

In the fall of 2012, as lawmakers and regulators began raising more red flags over the dangers of energy drinks and energy shots, *CBS Evening News* interviewed Manoj Bhargava, the man who became a billionaire by developing and marketing 5-hour Energy. When CBS correspondent Dr. Jon LaPook asked Bhargava what is in 5-hour Energy, he replied, "Amino acids are the main ingredients, and there's some caffeine."

"How much caffeine?"

"About as much as a medium Starbucks."

There was no reason for Bhargava to be coy about this. Like NVE's 6 Hour Power, like Coca-Cola and Monster, his company precisely calibrates the dose of powdered caffeine before blending it into beverages. Consumer Reports has even analyzed the caffeine contents of 5-hour Energy and found that it contains 215 milligrams (three SCADs) per shot, about as much as a twelve-ounce cup of Starbucks coffee. But Bhargava was following a long tradition of muddying the waters through analogies to coffee and imprecise labeling.

CHAPTER 15

Behind the Label

O n a crisp, sunny December day in 2011, Amelia Arria peered into a cooler at a 7-Eleven in College Park, Maryland. She perused the myriad energy drinks, each with its own, often inscrutable style of labeling. She pulled out a can of Monster Assault and showed me the label, which listed only a "proprietary energy blend" that included caffeine. A consumer would have no way of knowing how much caffeine the can contained.

Arria is the director of the Center on Young Adult Health and Development at the University of Maryland School of Public Health. She sort of stumbled onto energy drinks inadvertently. As she was interviewing college students for a long-term study, she was surprised to find that about half of them used energy drinks. She quickly learned there was a dearth of research in energy drinks. It was a totally new area of public health study.

I was visiting College Park to better understand the energy drink market and, in particular, the regulatory vacuum surrounding the products. We had strolled a couple hundred yards from Arria's office to the 7-Eleven to look at the energy drinks and talk to some customers. As in most modern convenience stores, wherever we stood we could reach out and grab a caffeine delivery mechanism—energy shots by the counter, colas stacked up along the aisles, caffeine tablets in the aisle with other over-the-counter medications, a large counter featuring several varieties of coffee, and a cooler taking up an entire wall, chockablock with caffeinated colas, energy drinks, and canned coffee products. Convenience stores are modern monuments to our lust for caffeine.

Most people we talked to seemed to have little idea how much caffeine each energy drink contained. One young man buying an energy drink called Xtreme Shock seemed to take umbrage at my inquiry. "Yeah, I know how much is in it," he said with slight disgust. "It's, like, 200 percent. It's, like, two cups of coffee. So yeah, I read the labels." Arria told me that many consumers have no idea how much caffeine is in the numerous new energy products, because the FDA does not require quantitative caffeine labeling—the bare minimum of information we need to make informed choices about appropriate doses. (Even soft drinks do not have to list the amount of caffeine they contain, but in 2007 Coca-Cola and Pepsi quietly announced that they would begin listing caffeine content per serving in soft drinks.)

In 2011, Arria and Mary Claire O'Brien, the doctor who was a critic of Four Loko, wrote a column in *The Journal of the American Medical Association*, listing concerns about energy drinks' effects on sleep, blood pressure, and patterns of addiction, and their use in cocktails. They also called for better labeling. "We thought that it would be a good idea for the consumers to actually know how much caffeine they were consuming," Arria told me. She wants to see warning labels, at least for caffeine-sensitive individuals and pregnant women, and an FDA-imposed caffeine limit for energy drinks.

Around the same time I interviewed Arria, the American Beverage Association drafted guidelines for energy drinks. In its "Guidance for the Responsible Labeling and Marketing of Energy Drinks," the ABA wrote, "Labels of energy drinks should follow ABA's established voluntary format for the labeling of caffeine and identify the quantity of caffeine from all sources contained in the beverage, for example, 'caffeine content xx mg/8 fl. oz.'" And it suggested specific wording for sensitive groups: "Labels of energy drinks should include the advisory statement 'Not (intended/recommended) for children, pregnant or nursing women (and/or persons/those) sensitive to caffeine.'"

The ABA also suggested energy drinks not be marketed in schools and that producers should not promote mixing energy drinks with alcohol. But adherence to these guidelines, it made clear, is entirely voluntary.

In response to several inquiries, ABA spokesperson Tracey Halliday sent me a statement about caffeine labeling. "Our industry's beverages are always labeled according to FDA regulations and, in many cases, go beyond what is required by law. Caffeine labeling is one example. In fact, in being responsive to consumers, many of our member companies have voluntarily placed caffeine amounts on beverage labels for several years," she wrote. "Consumers can find a wealth of information about what they're consuming by simply reading the labels on the foods and beverages they choose. When it comes to energy drinks, those who suggest they are not regulated by the FDA are simply spreading reckless misinformation."

Arria was heartened by the voluntary labeling effort, but feels the industry still has a long way to go. "They have better labels on grass seed than on energy drinks," she said.

⚡

After visiting the 7-Eleven, I went to see Susan Carlson, an FDA expert on caffeine regulations. Her office happens to be just a couple of miles from Arria's, in the large office park housing the FDA's Center for Food Safety and Applied Nutrition (CFSAN). Both women are PhD scientists, both are keenly interested in caffeine, and they both work in College Park. Although they knew of one another, they had never met. I pictured them passing in their cars in front of the 7-Eleven.

Carlson is a general health scientist in the office of food additive safety in CFSAN. Before we started talking about energy drink labeling, she made one thing clear: the FDA had yet to even draft a regulatory definition for energy drinks.

Complicating things further, some energy drinks are marketed as foods and some as beverages. In preparation for our interview, I brought some energy drinks along in a plain brown bag. The Red Bull in my bag had a "Nutrition Facts" label, putting it squarely in the food category. But I also had a can of Rockstar Roasted—an energy drink with added coffee—and it carried a "Supplement Facts" label, meaning it was regulated not as a food, but as a dietary supplement under the Dietary Supplement Health and Education Act of 1994 (DSHEA). And for good measure, I brought a can of Starbucks Doubleshot Energy—a coffee drink juiced with added caffeine—which is marketed as a food, even though it is racked right next to the Rockstar Roasted on cooler shelves.

Carlson said the FDA produced a document in 2009 designed to clear up the distinction between dietary supplements and beverages. It included this statement: "The packaging of liquid products in bottles or cans similar to those in which single or multiple servings of beverages like soda, bottled water, fruit juices, and iced tea are sold, suggests that the liquid product is intended for use as a conventional food."

Put another way, Rockstar and Monster and Amp and many other energy drinks were being marketed improperly. But when I asked Carlson about this, she said that they were not actually violating any FDA rule or regulation. "It's guidance," she said of the 2009 document, "so that means it's voluntary."

Carlson said the FDA's only caffeine regulation is the two hundred parts per million GRAS standard. I still did not understand how a bottler could legally exceed the caffeine concentration in the GRAS standard, but she explained that if a manufacturer exceeds that standard, it has to prove to the FDA that the product is safe.

In other words, if you want to market a caffeinated cola, you will not have to prove the caffeine is safe if you keep the concentration below that 200 parts per million GRAS standard. If your cola exceeds that caffeine concentration, you are, in essence, freestyling. You might be OK, but the onus is on you to prove that your product is safe. And even if an energy drink or juice includes caffeine at a level below the GRAS standard, it is reasonable to ask if the standard would apply to drinks other than colas, such as Mountain Dew or Sunkist.

When I left, I gave Carlson my bag full of drinks. The market was changing so quickly that there were several she had not seen before my visit.

By 2010, caffeine had become controversial in Canada, too, and Canadian bottlers were starting to feel the heat. The *Canadian Medical Association Journal* published an editorial advocating energy drink regulation. "Energy drinks are very effective high-concentration caffeine delivery systems," the editors wrote. They also said, "Caffeine-loaded energy drinks have now crossed the line from beverages to drugs delivered as tasty syrups."

While the FDA was taking a sort of laissez-faire approach to caffeine, Canadian regulators were getting the job done. Starting in 2013, regulations required that energy drinks not exceed 180 milligrams of caffeine per serving. Further, the products are to be sold as food, not dietary supplements, with caffeine contents clearly marked. And the drinks must have warning labels cautioning against mixing them with alcohol and stating that they are not suited for children, pregnant or breast-feeding women, and people sensitive to caffeine.

These regulations came in the wake of Canada's earlier regulations on caffeine in soft drinks, which restrict caffeine to 200 parts per million in cola-type beverages (this parallels the FDA's GRAS standard) and 150 parts per million for other caffeinated soft drinks, like Mountain Dew. Canada also disallows adding caffeine to juices or noncarbonated drinks.

In essence, Health Canada managed to regulate caffeine just as advocates in the United States kept hoping the FDA would. It's interesting to know that the panel appointed to look into this had recommended going much further: They wanted energy drinks to be renamed "stimulant drug containing drinks"; recommended a limit of 80 milligrams per serving; and said Health Canada should restrict their use to adults only, as with alcohol.

The European Union, too, has established its own set of regulations, requiring any beverages with more than 150 milligrams of caffeine per liter to be labeled with the words "high caffeine content," as well as the quantity of caffeine. And all of this information can't be buried on the back of the can, says the EU: "This wording must appear in the same field of vision as the name of the drink."

Meanwhile, the critique of energy drinks continues in the United States. In 2011, the American Academy of Pediatrics published a report that came to this conclusion: "Rigorous review and analysis of the literature reveal that caffeine and other stimulant substances contained in energy drinks have no place in the diet of children and adolescents."

It's clear that regulatory efforts on the federal level in the United States have been spotty, but things haven't fared much better at the local level. The University of New Hampshire wins the award for the most transitory effort to rein in energy drinks. On September 15, 2011, David May, the assistant vice president of business affairs, announced that energy drinks would be off campus store shelves by January, citing health concerns. "Just recently there was an incident on campus involving energy drinks that helped send a student to the hospital," he said in a press release.

Red Bull North America CEO Stefan Kozak responded with a letter, requesting a meeting with UNH president Mark Huddleston. Kozak noted, "Red Bull is now widely consumed in over 160 countries.

Last year alone, more than four billion cans and bottles were consumed worldwide, with about 1.5 billion of such cans in the US. Red Bull contains 80 mg caffeine per 8.4 oz. can, less than the amount of caffeine in one cup of coffee. Red Bull labels clearly and voluntarily label this amount."

President Huddleston replied with a letter to Kozak a week later, on September 30. "Thank you for your letter concerning our contemplated ban on the sale of energy drinks at dining and vending locations at the University of New Hampshire. In fact, I have concluded that we will continue sales of certain energy drinks, based on student interest, and the lack of clear evidence of patterns of abuse among our students. We are making this recommendation today." And with that, the two weeks of uncertainty were over. Red Bull remained on the shelves in Durham.

Soon enough, though, caffeinated energy products started catching heat from elected officials.

In February 2012, at the behest of Senator Chuck Schumer, the FDA sent a warning letter to the company that makes the caffeine inhalers known as AeroShots. These are lipstick-shaped plastic tubes developed by Harvard professor David Edwards. They are filled with one hundred milligrams of finely powdered caffeine and B vitamins. Edwards is a polymath who writes fiction and runs an art and design center in Paris named Le Laboratoire. An earlier creation of his, called Le Whif, was a similar delivery system for flavors like chocolate and was billed as "breathable food." But inhaling flavors is one thing; inhaling drugs yet another.

The FDA noted that AeroShot's promotional materials called it a caffeine inhaler. "Despite these suggestions that your product is intended for inhalation, you indicate in other statements that the product is intended for ingestion." The FDA said that dietary supplements must be intended for ingestion and that the AeroShot labeling is false and misleading because the "product cannot be intended for both inhalation and ingestion."

Then, in April, Illinois senator Dick Durbin asked FDA commissioner Margaret Hamburg to regulate energy drinks. In a letter to Hamburg, Durbin said he was concerned about the way the drinks are marketed toward young people. He wrote, "The website for Monster Energy Drink claims to deliver 'twice the buzz of a regular energy drink . . . and the big bad buzz you know and love.'"

Meanwhile, energy drinks continued to be marketed as a food but labeled as a supplement. In May 2012, the FDA did issue a warning letter to an energy drink bottler, but not over caffeine. In a letter addressed to Rockstar Energy Drink CEO Russell Weiner, the FDA said that a January 3, 2012, inspection of its manufacturing facility in Tennessee found labeling problems with the line of coffee-flavored energy products marketed under the Rockstar Roasted label. First of all, they were labeled as supplements, despite being marketed as a beverage. And the FDA noted an unapproved ingredient: not excessive caffeine, but ginkgo biloba leaf extract.

Weiner is another interesting caffeine entrepreneur. He trades mansions more often than most men buy shirts and brings to mind a younger Hugh Hefner, often using his houses in Hollywood and Miami to host flashy parties and photo shoots of bikini models. To a certain contingent of American men—the sort who read lad mags—Weiner is an aspirational figure. With his bling, conspicuous consumption, and models, he is the antithesis of the salt-of-the-earth Juan Valdez character.

Weiner's success did not come early. By the time he turned thirty in 2000, he had taken two runs at the California assembly and lost. He had cofounded the conservative Paul Revere Society with his father—Michael Savage, the ethnobotanist turned shock jock—but nobody noticed. He studied health food and herbs in Chicago. Then he helped a California entrepreneur produce a reduced-sugar cola. It flopped, badly. But Weiner had another trick up his sleeve. After having taken note of Red Bull's success, he launched Rockstar Energy Drink in 2001.

Weiner was outspoken about his conservative principles in Rockstar's early days. Though he has since toned it down, the company has faced boycotts from gay and lesbian groups due to its association with the emphatically antigay Savage. Despite this, Weiner has placed Rockstar firmly into the mainstream. In 2009, he left a distribution deal with Coke to join Pepsi, and in 2010, Rockstar sales rose 20 percent to forty-four million cases. (If you are counting, that includes 175,000 pounds of the bitter white powder that packs Rockstar's punch.) Like Monster and Red Bull, Rockstar is a billion-dollar brand.

Back to the FDA's 2012 letter. It asked Rockstar to relabel the energy drinks as conventional foods and remove the ginkgo from the formula. That July, an FDA employee went to the bottling plant to witness the company destroy its remaining ginkgo-infused product (it was allowed to export some of the product it had already canned). But the whole issue was not resolved until December.

On December 5, 2012, almost exactly a year after I'd interviewed Susan Carlson at the FDA's Center for Food Safety and Applied Nutrition, in College Park, Maryland, she took part in a meeting to resolve the FDA's concerns over Rockstar's coffee-flavored energy drinks. Rockstar sent three people to represent its interests: Ricardo Carvajal and Diane McColl, of Hyman, Phelps & McNamara, which claims to be the nation's largest food and drug law firm; and Larry McGirr, who had come from Canada on behalf of the multinational product-testing firm Intertek Cantox. The other team had more players on the field. In an indication of the FDA's increasing interest in energy products, no fewer than fifteen FDA regulators, scientists, and attorneys showed up or listened in via conference call. In the end, Rockstar agreed to label its energy drinks as food, not dietary supplements. Within months, Monster agreed to do the same.

By then, pressure on the energy drink companies had been growing for months.

In the summer of 2012, New York state attorney general Eric Schneiderman sent subpoenas to Monster, 5-hour Energy, and Pepsi, which bottles Amp. Schneiderman sought information about deceptive marketing claims and inaccurate labeling.

In August, FDA assistant commissioner for legislation Jeanne Ireland responded to Durbin's concerns with a five-page letter, basically saying that she was on it. The letter noted the guidance on distinguishing dietary supplements from foods. And it mentioned its warning to Rockstar's Weiner. It also mentioned a death that was getting some attention.

"Finally, to provide an update regarding the untimely death of Ms. Anais Fournier, as Commissioner Hamburg noted in her letter to you of May, 16, 2012, FDA did receive a Serious Adverse Event Report from the marketer of Monster Energy Drink," Ireland wrote. "We also received a voluntary Adverse Event Report from Ms. Fournier's family."

Adverse event reports are voluntary consumer complaints collected by the FDA's Center for Food Safety and Applied Nutrition. They are by no means comprehensive. For one thing, as the FDA says, they "only reflect information as reported and do not represent any conclusion by FDA about whether the product actually caused the actual events."

Fournier, a fourteen-year-old from Hagerstown, Maryland, drank a twenty-four-ounce Monster on December 16, 2011. The next evening, with her friends at the Valley Mall in Hagerstown, she drank another twenty-four-ounce can of Monster Energy, bought from a candy store. Each can contained 240 milligrams of caffeine (three SCADs). These twenty-four-ounce Monsters are big honkers. There's one product, called Mega Monster Energy, that is a screw-top can. And another, with a regular pop-top, called Monster Energy "BFC," which the teens know as a cruder variant of "big friggin' can."

A few hours after leaving the mall, Fournier was at home watching a movie with her family, when she went into cardiac arrest and fell unconscious. At the hospital, doctors put her into a medically induced coma. Six days later, at Johns Hopkins Hospital, doctors removed her from life support, and she died. The coroner listed the cause of death as "cardiac arrhythmia due to caffeine toxicity complicating mitral valve regulation in the setting of Ehlers-Danlos syndrome."

This was not the first death to be publicly associated with energy drinks and shots. The deaths of Toronto teen Brian Shepherd, after drinking Red Bull in 2008, and Antonio Hassell, who drank 5-hour Energy shots in Memphis in 2010, had also seen some press coverage. But Fournier's death got more attention, perhaps because she was a teenage girl, perhaps because her death came at a time when energy drinks were under greater scrutiny.

In November 2012, after the *New York Times* began reporting on adverse events associated with energy drinks and energy shots, the FDA released a comprehensive list of nearly eight years of adverse event reports related to Monster, Rockstar, and 5-hour Energy products. It was a scary list of ninety-three events, including thirteen deaths. Again, there is no way of knowing whether the energy products caused the deaths, but it was enough to scare the public and prompt the FDA to announce an investigation.

In a cover letter accompanying the adverse event reports, the agency included this warning: "FDA advises consumers to talk with their health care providers before using any product marketed as an 'energy shot' or 'energy drink.'" This seemed notable—dramatic, even—particularly considering the fact that the agency does not recommend checking with physicians before drinking colas or coffee.

It is hard to unravel the health problems attributed to energy drinks. Caffeine is not as powerful as cocaine, which can be deadly at just over a gram in naive users. But neither is it weak. For adults, ten grams—about a tablespoon—has long been considered a lethal dose. Some say it might be half that amount. Not that it's easy to consume that much. To take five grams of caffeine an adult would need to slam about sixteen 16-ounce cups of Starbucks coffee at once, or a hundred cups of tea. The newer products make overdose a little easier by concentrating the caffeine, but it's still not easy. Most adults would have to chug twenty to forty cans of Rockstar 2X Energy (with 250 milligrams of caffeine per can) to take that amount of caffeine.

Any of us who use caffeine eventually take more than we want to and might experience the sensation of a pounding heart, among other unpleasant effects. One young man who tried an energy shot told me, "I felt like I was going to have a heart attack." It might feel that way, but a bit too much caffeine will not likely harm your heart.

Even among those people with arrhythmias—disorders that cause the heart to beat too fast, too slow, or irregularly—caffeine does little harm. A 2011 literature review published in *The American Journal of Medicine* found no reason for concern. "With the conflicting data that are available, it is understandable that most physicians are unsure of the advice they can provide about caffeine intake and arrhythmias," Daniel Pelchovitz and Jeffrey Goldberger wrote. "A common idea in practice is that caffeine intake should be limited in patients at risk for arrhythmia; however, it is unclear what evidence provides support for this."

The authors concluded that "in most patients with known or suspected arrhythmia, caffeine in moderate doses is well tolerated and there is therefore no reason to restrict ingestion of caffeine." It would be easy to be skeptical of this finding. First off, Goldberger is a consultant for Red Bull. And there is the sense that caffeine can feel so hard on the heart. But despite numerous studies, doctors have been unable to find a link between moderate caffeine use and heart disease or disturbance in most people. However, recent research does suggest an association between coffee and nonfatal heart attacks in people with a genetic predisposition to metabolize caffeine slowly.

Other health concerns are far less severe, but far more numerous: A 2011 report showed that emergency room visits related to energy drinks increased tenfold between 2005 and 2009. An update of that report, published in 2013, showed that ER visits doubled from 10,068 in 2007 to 20,783 in 2011. Males were more apt to get into trouble with the drinks than females, and the eighteen-to-twenty-five age group was most commonly involved. The report, from the federal Drug Abuse Warning Network, found that most ER visits involved energy drinks alone, but a significant number included bad interactions with drugs: 27 percent with pharmaceuticals (and a third of those involved other central nervous system stimulants, like Ritalin and Adderall); 13 percent involved alcohol (these are the problems that came to a head with Four Loko); and 5 percent involved marijuana.

Monster was quick to respond, in a press release adorned with its neon green claw-mark logo: "The DAWN report also misleadingly compared the caffeine content in energy drinks with that in a 5-ounce cup of coffee. The vast majority of coffee drinks are consumed in sizes substantially larger than 5 ounces and contain caffeine levels similar to, and in many cases higher than, energy drinks. In fact, the leading brands of coffeehouse-brewed coffee typically contain more than 20 mg of caffeine per ounce, which means a medium 16-ounce coffeehouse coffee contains at least 320 mg of caffeine."

Monster may have slightly overstated the caffeine levels of coffeehouse coffee, but that's a quibble. In terms of caffeine, it would be safe to assume that if a dose of 240 milligrams of caffeine, which Fournier consumed, could kill a person, then Starbucks would have seen at least a few deaths from their coffee, which might contain this amount of caffeine in a twelve- or sixteen-ounce cup. But of the forty-one adverse event reports the FDA received for Starbucks coffee in the same eight-year period as the energy drinks and shots that caused so much concern (when there were ninety-three reports for 5-hour Energy and forty for Monster), just a few required emergency room visits. However, one report detailed a cardiac event that required hospitalization, and it sounded scary ("tachyarrhythmia, blood caffeine increased, cardiac enzymes increased, troponin I increased, myocardial infarction").

So what might account for Fournier's death? And what might account for the other health problems attributed to energy drinks?

The first is the pattern doctors call "true, true, and unrelated." A person might drink energy drinks and then have a heart problem—true and true—but did the former cause the latter, or are they unrelated? The perception that there might be a relationship leads to what doctors call "ascertainment bias," or "sampling bias," which occurs anytime a subgroup is overrepresented in a data set, skewing the results. In the case of caffeine, it might be that people who suffer a heart attack after drinking an energy shot or energy drink are more likely to associate the heart trouble with the product than are people who suffer heart attacks after drinking coffee. It would be a simple explanation, and one that could hold some appeal for the energy drink industry. But in Fournier's case, there was the coroner's report listing caffeine toxicity as the cause of death.

Another faint, but scary, possibility is that there's some energy drink component that is toxic when ingested with caffeine. This was the problem with ephedra. Scientists say more research is needed, but there are hints that something beyond caffeine may be causing health problems associated with energy drinks.

There are accounts suggesting that heavy use of energy drinks could cause strokes or seizures in some people. A pair of Arizona neurologists reported on four patients who had seizures after heavy energy drink consumption. One man had a seizure after drinking two 24-ounce Rockstars quickly on an empty stomach. And a woman showed up in the emergency room after drinking a 24-ounce Monster on top of the caffeine-based diet pills she was taking. In all cases, the patients seemed fine without energy drinks. "Once the patients were abstinent from the energy drinks, no recurrent seizures were reported," the doctors wrote. "We propose that the large consumption of energy drinks rich in caffeine, taurine and guarana seed extract could have provoked the seizures." Other individual reports of seizures associated with energy drinks come from Italy and Turkey.

Another strange case comes from Australia. A twenty-eight-year-old suffered cardiac arrest after a long day of motocross racing and chugging Red Bulls. He'd had seven or eight cans of Red Bull over seven hours. That sounds like a lot. But it is just 640 milligrams of caffeine—about a tenth of the amount considered a lethal dose. The authors suggested that the combination of strenuous exercise and caffeine and taurine (an additive to Red Bull and many other energy drinks) might lead to fatal heart attacks in some people.

On October 17, 2012, a team of attorneys filed a civil action with the Riverside County Superior Court of California. It was titled "Wendy Crossland and Richard Fournier; individually and as surviving parents of Anais Fournier v. Monster Beverage Corporation."

The case contained seven complaints, including negligence and wrongful death. The take-home message was this: "Defendant's failures in designing, manufacturing, marketing, distribution, warning and/or selling MONSTER ENERGY drinks directly and proximately caused Anais Fournier to suffer the cardiac arrhythmia that ultimately led to her death."

The lawyers sent out a press release, quoting Fournier's mother. "I was shocked to learn the FDA can regulate caffeine in a can of soda, but not these huge energy drinks," Wendy Crossland said. "With their bright colors and names like Monster, Rockstar, and Full Throttle, these drinks are targeting teenagers with no oversight or accountability. These drinks are death traps for young, developing girls and boys, like my daughter Anais."

On November 15, sandwiched between testimony on Superstorm Sandy and UN Ambassador Susan Rice's role in the attacks on a U.S. Embassy in Libya, Senators Durbin and Blumenthal took to the floor to call for better regulation of the energy drink industry and mentioned Fournier.

Monster responded with a press release questioning the medical evidence. It claimed that Fournier regularly drank energy drinks and Starbucks coffee. It said the autopsy report of caffeine toxicity was based only on Fournier's mother's report of her drinking an energy drink, not on a blood test. And it detailed her heart conditions, including Ehlers-Danlos syndrome, intramural coronary artery thickening, and myocardial fibrosis.

If nothing else, the Fournier case was becoming a full-blown PR disaster for Monster. And the company had related problems running on a parallel track. Starting in spring 2012, investors began wondering if the stock of the publicly traded company was overpriced. In April, the *Wall Street Journal* had reported that Coca-Cola was in talks to buy Monster, which it already distributed in some areas. But that report caused the price to jump, and Coke to walk, according to the newspaper.

By that summer, some hedge funds were smelling blood. Robert MacArthur, of Alternative Research Services, a Connecticut firm that conducts research for hedge funds, was sending out regular twenty-page missives collating all of the available anti–energy drink information.

Investors were, indeed, growing wary. By early November, in its third-quarter earnings call, Monster's Rodney Sacks led with the concerns about the drink's safety and its regulatory status. He even got into the arcana of labeling. "Another area of recent media focus has been on the fact that Monster Energy drinks are labeled as dietary supplement rather than as foods. In the case of Monster Energy drinks, this is a red herring. Our products could be labeled and sold as foods if we chose to do so."

And Sacks used the coffee analogy, telling investors, "a 16-ounce can of Monster Energy contains about half the caffeine of a 16-ounce cup of coffee-house brew coffee; even a 24-ounce can of Monster Energy, which contains about 240 milligrams of caffeine from all sources, has about 30 percent less caffeine than an average, medium-sized 16-ounce cup of coffee house brew coffee. . . . Even an extra large–sized serving of Mountain Dew fountain drink, which is readily available throughout America, contains about 234 milligrams of caffeine."

But Sacks had good news to report: Third-quarter gross sales had hit a record high of $632 million.

By May 2013, Monster was facing another adversary in court. This time it was San Francisco city attorney Dennis Herrera, who accused Monster of unfair, deceptive, and unlawful business practices. Herrera listed a number of health concerns and said Monster had made unsubstantiated claims about its "energy blend," when caffeine is really carrying all the freight. But mostly, he said, Monster was marketing its drinks to kids. "Despite the dangers to youth of consuming energy drinks and MONSTER's own warning label which acknowledges these risks, MONSTER aggressively markets its products to children and teenagers by sponsoring youth sports tournaments and prominently featuring profiles of youth ranging in age from 6 to 17 on its Monster Army website," the suit asserts. "MONSTER also targets children and teenagers by promoting a 'lifestyle' that features extreme sports, music, gaming, military themes, and the scantily-clad 'Monster Girls.' As a direct result of MONSTER's targeted advertising efforts, its products are popular with and frequently consumed by youth."

In June 2013, energy drink marketing also caught the attention of the American Medical Association. At a policy meeting, the AMA supported a ban of the marketing of high stimulant/caffeine drinks to adolescents under the age of eighteen.

For its part, Monster hired a doctor with a familiar face to carry its water. Bob Arnot, an athletic man once known as "Dr. Sport," has served as a medical correspondent for CBS and NBC, hosted the cable show *Dr. Danger*, and has written books on health.

While Monster was facing growing pressure from its critics, the coffee industry was feeling pressure from Monster and its ilk. For one thing, energy drinks had actually surpassed coffee as the favorite source of caffeine among one select demographic group.

When Harris Lieberman and his colleagues set out to investigate caffeine use among active-duty army soldiers in 2007, they did not know what to expect. For generations, coffee had been a soldier's best friend. As that 1896 report pointed out, "the American soldier, with but few exceptions, wants coffee, and plenty of it," but things appeared to be changing fast.

Lieberman's team surveyed 990 soldiers on nine U.S. bases and two overseas sites. The researchers asked the subjects how often they used any of dozens of caffeinated products, asking forty-three more questions to understand the soldiers' demographic information and dietary habits.

Some results were not surprising. For example, 82 percent of the soldiers used at least one caffeinated product daily, which is about what we expect of most American adults. Among regular caffeine users, men took 365 milligrams daily (nearly five SCADs) and women took 216 (about three SCADs).

Coffee was still the most prevalent caffeine delivery mechanism, followed by soft drinks. And hot tea was hardly a blip on the screen; bottled teas were twice as popular. So far, no surprises. "Coffee was the largest single source of caffeine intake for both males and females," they reported, "and energy beverages were the second highest contributor to intake of regular caffeine consumers of both sexes, with male consumption more than four times that of females."

Here's where it gets interesting. While both male and female soldiers drank sodas more often than energy drinks, the men were getting more caffeine overall from the energy drinks. (It's not really a surprise that men use more energy drinks than women, given that the bottlers target that demographic heavily. The bikini models, action-sports events, and heavy metal music are all geared toward them.) Lieberman also found that energy drinks had actually passed coffee among one group of those surveyed. The older soldiers are still drinking more coffee and taking more caffeine than the young males. But the young men, those soldiers from eighteen to twenty-four, get more caffeine from energy drinks than coffee.

Here we have the retort to those who claim that energy drinks will never replace coffee: For some Americans, they already have.

CHAPTER 16

Showdown

⚡

On May 1, 2013, a gaggle of food-industry honchos rushed in to see Michael Taylor, the FDA's deputy commissioner for foods and veterinary medicine. There was Casey Keller, from Wrigley; Brad Figel, Matthias Berninger, and John Luedke, from Mars Inc., the global food giant that owns Wrigley; and Stuart Pape, from the legal and lobbying firm Patton Boggs, which has represented the soft drink industry before the FDA for years.

If they looked nervous, they had good reason. On April 29, Taylor had announced the agency would be investigating the safety of adding caffeine to food products for the first time since 1980. "The only time that FDA explicitly approved the added use of caffeine in a food was for cola and that was in the 1950s," Taylor said in his statement. "Today, the environment has changed. Children and adolescents may be exposed to caffeine beyond those foods in which caffeine is naturally found and beyond anything FDA envisioned when it made the determination regarding caffeine in cola."

Surprisingly, the item that finally spurred the FDA into action was not any of the more extreme energy products, not the gel strips LeBron James was promoting, not even the 5-hour Energy shots that

Jerry Seinfeld once called "meth-lab, Hawaiian Punch Jell-O shots." It was gum.

In April, Wrigley had introduced Alert Energy Caffeine Gum. It got a lot of attention, and Wrigley promoted it well. Aiming to appeal to the omnivorous caffeine enthusiasts among us, Wrigley partnered with 7-Eleven for an ad in *USA Today*, which ran this copy: "Here are two new ways to perk up your day. Swing by 7-Eleven for a cup of our new Skinny Salted Caramel Mocha, and you'll get a free pack of ALERT ENERGY Caffeine Gum."

Caffeinated gum is nothing new. Jolt gum was introduced in 2004. By 2013, civilians could buy the same Stay Alert used for military rations (though it changed its name to Military Energy Gum concurrent with the Wrigley gum launch). And Java Gum has played on concerns about the safety of Monster Energy with its tagline: "Don't be afraid, we're no monster."

One problem with caffeinated gum is that it can be easily confused with its drug-free cousins. In May 2011, more than six hundred students at a primary school in South Africa fell ill after chewing Blitz Caffeine Energy Gum. The gum had been recovered from a nearby farm, where it had been dumped because its expiration date had passed.

In any case, it was the gum that finally nudged the FDA into action. Taylor made his announcement on a Monday. By Wednesday the delegation from Wrigley and Mars had come to meet with Taylor. And one week later, on May 8, Wrigley said it was pulling the product from the market.

"After discussions with the FDA, we have a greater appreciation for its concern about the proliferation of caffeine in the nation's food supply," Wrigley announced. "There is a need for changes in the regulatory framework to better guide the consumers and the industry about the appropriate level and use of caffeinated products. In an effort to support this process, and out of respect for the FDA, we have paused the production, sales, and marketing of *Alert*."

Taylor applauded the decision, saying, "We hope others in the food industry will exercise similar restraint."

But in the caffeine delivery mechanism industry, there did not seem to be much restraint going around. It wasn't just that the FDA was closing the door after the horses had left the barn; the horses were running roughshod through a regulatory Wild West. Corralling caffeine at that point made putting toothpaste back in the tube look pretty easy.

And the caffeine industry was taking a keen interest in the FDA's new initiative. Two weeks after Wrigley pulled its gum off the shelves, another food industry delegation arrived to meet with Taylor. The American Beverage Association sent a posse of five: Jim McGreevy, Tracey Halliday, Susan Neely, Patti Vaughan, and Dick Adamson. Mars Inc.'s David Kamenetzky showed up. And Stuart Pape came back for more. While Taylor had not mentioned soft drinks as a target of his investigation, the association represents energy drink bottlers like Monster, Red Bull, and Rockstar. It also represents Coca-Cola, which not only distributes Monster but bottles its own NOS and Full Throttle energy drinks, and Pepsi, which distributes Rockstar and bottles Amp. And, of course, ABA is closely watching any regulations pertaining to powdered caffeine, because its members use millions of pounds of the stuff annually.

A month after Wrigley pulled its gum, and a few weeks after the delegation from the American Beverage Association crowded the room, I went to Maryland to interview Taylor at the FDA's large White Oak campus. Friendly but businesslike, he told me he had two parallel concerns, saying that the new energy products have broken out of the typical boundaries around caffeine and are a far cry from the traditional coffee, tea, and chocolate. And in the process, the food industry is flagrantly skirting food additive regulations.

"There are some fair questions to be asked from a public-health, consumer-protection vantage point before we go down this pathway much further," he said.

I mentioned that Red Bull had sort of nudged open the door, found some suitable habitat, and its imitators and successors had then flooded the zone. Taylor agreed that the process had been incremental. He said the industry could argue that energy drinks are an extension of the soft drink, or non-nutritive beverage, category, but with amped-up caffeine levels. "But then you see Campbell's having its V8 Fusion product—it's a healthy, nutritional product with caffeine, and intrinsically not hugely concerning, because it is a product that does not necessarily appeal to kids. But then you saw the next steps, toward solid foods, then toward different forms of delivery like the MiO Energy drops, and then you have the gum."

And he explained something that had puzzled me. Since caffeinated gum was not really new, why was it the product that finally spurred the FDA into action? He said it was partly a matter of scale. "We've seen a big shifting in the food category, from some sort-of fringy, small players doing this to some of the most iconic food companies in the country making these decisions," Taylor told me. "And one of our concerns was signaling that we need to sort of hold on here for a second to make sure we know what we are doing from a safety standpoint." So it is one thing if a smallish New Jersey company is producing a caffeinated gum under the Jolt brand and altogether another if an internationally recognized brand like Wrigley launches a similar product.

Taylor said the new products that are not quite energy drinks pose particular regulatory challenges. I had brought along a bag of CDMs, and I spread them out on the table before us. One was a small plastic vial with a squeeze top, looking a bit like the vials of food coloring often used to dye Easter eggs. It was MiO Energy, from the food giant Kraft. Here is how the company described the "liquid water enhancer" in a press release: "When added to water, MiO creates a vibrant swirl of color that self-mixes to create a delicious, personalized drink. . . . MiO Energy is a recent extension of MiO, but with an energy and B-vitamin benefit with 60 mg caffeine per 8 fluid ounce serving—about the same amount of caffeine as a 6 oz. cup of coffee." Kraft's TV ads call it "portable power on demand."

MiO is basically a slurry of caffeine powder and artificial flavor—a concentrated chemical stew. A 1.08-ounce vial contains 720 milligrams of caffeine (almost ten SCADs). It is creative, convenient, and it tastes fine when used as directed. In essence, the blend of chemical flavors and caffeine is similar to a super-concentrated diet soft drink. But it is not the sort of product the FDA anticipated when it established its caffeine standard in 1958. For one thing, it is easy for anyone to use the whole thing in one beverage, and many kids have posted online videos of themselves drinking a full vial in less than a minute. (Judging from the facial expressions, part of the challenge is the concentrated sour flavor.)

Just as Taylor announced the FDA's caffeine investigation, something else happened. The DSM-5, the 2013 revision of the American Psychiatric Association's diagnostic tome, landed with a resounding thump. This edition added the diagnosis of caffeine withdrawal syndrome that Roland Griffiths had long lobbied for (as mentioned in chapter 5), prompting a slew of news stories. One headline read, CRASHING ON CAFFEINE NOW A MENTAL DISORDER. While some had fun with the news, other stories paid close attention to caffeine withdrawal and how to deal with it. Suddenly, it seemed, caffeine was getting some long overdue attention and respect.

Meanwhile, there were a few subtle hints that people in the soft drink industry were starting—slowly, perhaps, and tentatively—to acknowledge caffeine's importance in their products. Or at least to acknowledge that their caffeinated products are stimulating. Wrigley deserves credit for putting the word *caffeine* right up front in its Alert Energy Caffeine Gum, however ill-fated the product launch was. In early 2013, Pepsi launched Kickstart. Calling it a "sparkling juice beverage," Pepsi's Greg Lyons said, "Our consumers told us they are looking for an alternative to traditional morning beverages—one that tastes great, includes real fruit juice, and has just the right amount of kick to help them start their days."

Notably, Pepsi does not hide Kickstart's caffeine; it put the word boldly on the front of the can, right next to its claim of 5 percent juice. Kickstart contains ninety-two milligrams of caffeine per sixteen-ounce can. Again, this is not an arbitrary level. Pepsi formulated Kickstart, like Pepsi Max, with a caffeine concentration just below the FDA's two hundred parts per million standard for caffeine.

Putting the word *caffeine* on the label hints at a subtle but significant shift on Pepsi's part, perhaps prompted by the increasing interest in energy drinks. Caffeine is stepping out of the shadows.

At a 2012 investors' symposium, Pepsi CFO Hugh Johnston detailed the company's "energy strategy." He mentioned Starbucks Refreshers as a new entry to the energy market, to bolster its own Amp brand and the Rockstar it distributes. Johnston also placed a caffeinated soft drink squarely in the energy category, something the industry has long resisted, saying Mountain Dew "was in many ways really the original energy drink." This is a big change in messaging from the 1980s, when Mountain Dew had the same concentration of caffeine as it does today but the industry claimed caffeine was just a flavor.

Pepsi had been trying to launch new caffeinated products for years, with limited success. In 1996 it marketed the pioneering energy drink Josta, caffeinated with guarana, but discontinued it by 1999. And its Pepsi Kona coffee drink sputtered, too, also in the mid-1990s.

But by 2012, Pepsi was on a roll. It announced that three products had passed the billion-dollar sales mark. Diet Mountain Dew, Brisk iced tea, and Starbucks ready-to-drink beverages brought the company to twenty-two billion-dollar brands. The three new additions—a diet soda, a tea, and a coffee drink—had just one thing in common: caffeine. They were in good company. The corporation's other billion-dollar brands with caffeine included Pepsi, Diet Pepsi, Pepsi Max, Mountain Dew, and Lipton.

Coca-Cola's billion-dollar brands, which contributed to its 2012 sales of $48 billion, included plenty of caffeine delivery mechanisms: Coca-Cola, Diet Coke, Coca-Cola Zero, and, in Japan, Ayataka bottled tea and Georgia canned coffee. Coca-Cola was also starting to break its silence on caffeine's psychoactive effects. The company's Minute Maid Enhanced juice drink noted on the label: "37–43 mg of natural caffeine per bottle for an energy lift." Again, this breaks the long-standing tradition of claiming that the levels of caffeine found in its colas—34 milligrams in 12 ounces of Coke; 46 milligrams in 12 ounces of Diet Coke—were just there for flavoring.

In 2013, Coca-Cola posted on its Web site a video of Dr. Sandra Fryhofer discussing the drug in a bit more depth. "Some caffeine is fine. It helps you wake up; it increases mental alertness. But too much can cause anxiety, nervousness, sleep problems, elevated blood pressure, heart palpitations, and muscle tremors."

It is a video clearly intended to mark Coca-Cola's position on energy drinks for young people, with Fryhofer stating that children from four to twelve should have no more than 45 to 85 milligrams of caffeine daily. (This could actually be a hell of a lot—a 45-pound six-year-old taking 75 milligrams is the same as a 180-pound adult taking 4 SCADs.) "But one thing is clear," Fryhofer concluded. "Highly caffeinated energy drinks have no place in the diets of adolescents and children."

$$\large \mathcal{\not{}}$$

Back at the FDA, I pulled another caffeine drink out of the bag I had brought with me to show Mike Taylor: a strange hybrid called Refreshers, developed by Starbucks.

Starbucks stands out among modern caffeine hucksters. It has developed an internationally recognized brand, a vast network of cafés, and a fast-growing line of ready-to-drink caffeinated beverages. It's got tea wrapped up, too, with its Tazo and Teavana lines (it spent $620 million for the latter in late 2012). It mass-markets roasted-and-ground coffees in supermarkets and has its lowbrow Seattle's Best Coffee in bags and cans. It developed its own proprietary coffee pod system; by early 2013, the Verismo machines were being offered at Starbucks stores for $199, along with four free boxes of pods.

And the coffee in Starbucks cafés, meanwhile, has continued to evolve away from its trademark dark roasts. The coffees it made its early reputation on were so uniformly dark roasted—burnt, even— that they earned the company the moniker "Charbucks." First, it introduced a medium-roast coffee called Pike Place Roast. Then, it developed an even lighter roast so mild all that seemingly remains is a caffeinated base for the cream and sugar. Or so you might think after reading Starbucks press materials: "To draw out its soft flavors, Starbucks Blonde Roast has a shorter roast time, creating a premium, approachable and perfectly balanced cup of lighter-bodied coffee that goes great with cream and sugar." To sweeten the pot, Starbucks began offering premixed Vanilla Blonde drinks—the light-roast coffee blended with vanilla syrup.

Starbucks has also approached the value-added, single-serving coffee from a less expected angle, by marketing instant coffee. Its Via "natural roasted instant and microground coffee" is an intriguing blend of the highbrow and low. It's got all of the flowery verbiage of other Starbucks coffees. ("Grown in Colombia's rich volcanic soil, this coffee is as distinctive as the countryside. Starbucks VIA Ready Brew Colombia delivers round body, juicy mouthfeel and signature nutty flavor—in an instant.") But it is not all talk—Starbucks does seems to have reduced, but not eliminated altogether, the sour flavor that has been a hallmark of instant coffees. (A barista once described it to me as the flavor of vomit, a disgusting but apt analogy.)

Via is so successful—you can even buy it in China, labeled in Mandarin—that Starbucks broke ground in 2012 on a 180,000-square-foot plant in Augusta, Georgia, with a capacity of cranking out 4,000 metric tons of instant coffee annually. To put that into perspective, each serving weighs but 3.3 grams. The plant will be able to produce more than a billion tubes of instant coffee in a year, each retailing for nearly a dollar. (We can only hope this will allow Augusta hotels to serve stronger coffee than the "rather weak infusion" that was on hand for the laudanum overdose victim in 1859.)

Moving from single-serving coffee products toward the energy drink market, Starbucks developed Refreshers. Launched in 2012, Starbucks Refreshers are energy drinks packaged in brightly colored cans. With this design, the antithesis of Monster's garish claw marks, it looks like the marketers are targeting women. Like their canned coffees, Starbucks produces them in partnership with Pepsi.

Launching the drinks, Starbucks said in a press release, "The introduction to the Starbucks Refreshers beverages brand platform is an evolution of the coffee market using a new breakthrough coffee experience using green coffee extract, resulting in thirst-quenching, delicious, low calorie refreshment with a boost of natural energy from caffeine and fruit juice." And with Refreshers, Starbucks is making a promise that sounds utterly bizarre for the company that brought bold, rich, dark-roasted coffee to the masses: "No coffee flavor. I promise," Starbucks's Brian Smith says on its Web site. "Just a refreshing break from the roasty norm."

So what is the "breakthrough coffee experience" in a sweet, carbonated beverage that tastes nothing like coffee? The only thing Refreshers have in common with Starbucks coffee is caffeine. With Refreshers, it has taken obfuscation to a new height, playing games with its wording. Each can of Refreshers promises "natural energy from green coffee extract," but the word *caffeine* appears nowhere on the label. Watching Starbucks perform logical and verbal gymnastics to leap around the word brings to mind Lily Tomlin's sentiment: No matter how cynical you get, it is impossible to keep up.

Bringing the evolution of Starbucks caffeine delivery mechanisms together, it is now selling its Refreshers in the little Via tubes. More conveniently packaged Starbucks caffeine for people who don't like coffee.

⚡

Among the CDMs I'd brought to Taylor's office was one that blurred the line between coffee and energy drinks: a discontinued K-Cup labeled "revv Pulse, with ginseng and guarana." When I showed it to him, he smiled and said, "You've got to hand it to the marketing people." He was right. In the spring of 2010, as Green Mountain launched revv and revv Pulse, it even registered the trademark "Nature's original energy drink," for its coffee and coffee-based beverages. Its press release read, "Responding to the exploding consumer interest in energy drinks, Green Mountain Coffee has introduced two new K-Cup portion packs for Keurig Single-Cup brewers that contain more coffee and more kick." The K-Cups are black with neon green highlights, a direct imitation of the Monster color scheme.

These products may seem foreign to coffee traditionalists, who prefer to think of their naturally caffeinated beverage in an altogether different category than the products enhanced with powdered caffeine. But they also point out some of caffeine's regulatory quirks. Before launching revv Pulse, Green Mountain asked the FDA if it could add powdered caffeine to K-Cups, to compensate for any caffeine lost in roasting. The agency's response? No, unless they could provide the science showing it was safe.

Green Mountain was undeterred. It wanted to boost its caffeine contents to get a piece of the fast-growing energy drink sector. So instead it boosted its K-Cups with ginseng and guarana. Since the FDA sometimes considers low levels of natural ingredients like guarana to be flavorings, Green Mountain appears to have skirted the agency's advice against boosting their coffee with straight caffeine powder. But Green Mountain discontinued the line without explanation in 2012.

Given the trends in the market, it's not hard to imagine the perfect caffeine delivery mechanism. It would have the rich coffee flavor most Americans love. It would come in convenient, prepackaged single-serving doses, like Coke and K-Cups. It would be sweet, like Coke and Monster. It would have plenty of caffeine, like coffee and energy drinks. But unlike coffee, the caffeine quantity would be consistent. It might look quite like a coffee-flavored energy drink.

Biologists use the phrase "convergent evolution" to describe two species that have started in completely different forms and developed similar traits in order to exploit the same niche. Dolphins and fish are one example; Java Monster and Starbucks Doubleshot, another.

The former began as an energy drink; the latter started life as a canned coffee. Java Monster evolved when a caffeinated energy drink was flavored with coffee. Starbucks Doubleshot evolved when a coffee drink was juiced with added caffeine (by the label, it's a "fortified energy coffee drink"). They occupy the same habitat in the cooler case, cheek by jowl. The ecological niche, the market demand, was there, and just a couple of evolutionary steps brought these drinks together, from different origins.

It is not just Monster and Starbucks that are competing in this Darwinian marketplace. Arizona Beverage Co. came at this from the tea side of things, to produce the energy drink Joltin' Joe. Rockstar Roasted boasts "premium blended latte & cream coffee," and is fortified with caffeine, guarana, ginseng, B vitamins, and taurine. The National Federation of Coffee Growers of Colombia even took a crack at this with Juan Valdez Double Kick (which seems to have gone extinct). These drinks are increasingly popular. Java Monster sales grew nearly 25 percent in the third quarter of 2012.

The beverage industry is not fumbling in the dark here; they are dialing in to optimal caffeination to keep consumers coming back. Consider the specificity of a 2005 coffee-drink patent from industry giant Nestlé. "Controlled Delivery of Caffeine from High-Caffeinated Coffee Beverages Made from Soluble Powder" details the steps for blending coffee powder and natural caffeine. And Nestlé described it in terms of the intended metabolic effect: "Thus, a beverage can be prepared that contains at least 80 to no more than 115 mg caffeine such that consumption of a single serving of the beverage by a person provides a plasma caffeine level in the person that is above 1.25 mg/l for at least 2 to 4 hours following consumption of the beverage." You read that right—the beverage formulators are blending caffeine powder and coffee with the goal of hitting your ideal "plasma caffeine level."

When I showed Taylor the can of Java Monster Mean Bean that I'd bought at a 7-Eleven that morning, he quickly looked at the label. "Caffeine is declared here in the context of an energy blend, but they don't give the quantitative information," he said. It was a reminder that although much had changed since my first visit to the FDA in 2011, some caffeine labeling was still lousy. A year and a half after the American Beverage Association had publicized its voluntary guidelines for energy drinks, and months after Monster had announced it would start labeling its energy drinks as foods and quantify the caffeine, this product was still marketed as a supplement, and its caffeine contents remained inscrutable.

Taylor drinks coffee and Diet Coke (sometimes caffeine-free), and he clearly understands the challenge of regulating caffeine and the limits regulators might face. "I got asked by somebody, 'Are we going to put age limits on coffee, so if you go to Starbucks would you have to show an ID?' I would consider that not realistic," he said. "Nobody's oblivious to the reality in which we live."

But he made a distinction between the more traditional uses of caffeine and the new breed of energy drinks. Holding the Monster, he said, "This is not a historic, cultural aspect of caffeine."

Java Monster may not seem historic and cultural, but it was inevitable. The surprise is not that caffeine delivery mechanisms evolved into these blends of flavoring chemicals and caffeine powder. The surprise is that it took so long. One man saw this trend coming a mile away and articulated it beautifully.

Emil Fischer is the German chemist who won a Nobel Prize in 1902, seven years after he pioneered the synthesis of caffeine in a lab. In a lecture that year, he predicted that factories would soon be synthesizing caffeine on a large scale, and this would reduce its cost. Of course, Fischer was right. The German factories began marketing synthetic caffeine within a few decades of his talk. The rest of these remarks now seem prophetic:

When it is considered that caffeine is the most active constituent of the two most widespread stimulants, coffee and tea, the matter takes on quite a different complexion. It is common knowledge that for a long time efforts have been made to replace those still rather costly substances by cheaper ones. The clearest proof is the large number of coffee substitutes which appear on the market. Nevertheless all these substitutes lack the best feature of coffee and tea, i.e. the pleasant stimulating effect that originates from the caffeine content. This shortcoming could readily be overcome by the addition of synthetic caffeine as soon as it has become cheap enough, and once this step has been taken, an improvement in the taste and aroma of those substitutes will not fail to follow. It is even possible to produce the true aroma of coffee or tea artificially, too, by synthesis; with the exercise of a little imagination the day can be foreseen when beans will no longer be required to make good coffee: a small amount of powder from a chemical works together with water will provide a savoury, refreshing drink surprisingly cheaply. The layman usually receives with scepticism such prophecies by the chemist and in this specific instance his scepticism will not be weakened by the knowledge that a constituent of guano would be used to prepare the synthetic drink.

Fischer was presaging a lot, even beyond the looming synthesis of caffeine on a commercial scale. He also anticipated the public's reluctance to take caffeine made from uric acid, which would be Coca-Cola's concern in the 1950s. Fischer's pince-nez must have been especially clear, because he even anticipated Java Monster, Rockstar Roasted, and their ilk. He was proposing just such beasts a century before their generation of coffee-flavored energy drinks. If the layman received the chemist's prophecy skeptically in 1902, he does no longer. We need only look to the nearest cooler for drinks with coffee flavor and "a small amount of powder from a chemical works."

The modern energy drinks look an awful lot like high-tech, gussied-up versions of Asa Candler's Coca-Cola. A century after the Chattanooga trial, the caffeine science is better, and the temperate Taylor is in the role once played by the bombastic Wiley. But the FDA is still wrestling with the same questions: Is caffeine addictive? Should it be treated differently when it is added to colas and energy drinks than when it is a natural constituent of coffee or tea? Is it healthy for children and adolescents? And how should the federal government regulate it?

⚡

The American Beverage Association, which seems to drop a press release whenever the soft drink industry comes in for criticism, was uncharacteristically mum after its delegation visited Taylor to talk about caffeine.

Michael Jacobson, the longtime advocate for caffeine regulation, told me he had not expected the FDA investigation. "I'm surprised," he said, "because it is so hard to get FDA to do anything."

Jacobson told me he is concerned that the FDA might study it to death before taking any regulatory action, and he will believe caffeine regulation when he sees it. He said, "The chicken way out would be just to require caffeine-content labeling," instead of doing that in addition to requiring warning labels on caffeinated beverages and establishing limits on the amounts of added caffeine.

Taylor said labeling is one of the regulatory options he might consider. Another would be setting enforceable caffeine limits. But he said he would not prejudge the FDA's investigation. "The mode we are in is first getting the science together."

As a first step, he asked the Institute of Medicine of the National Academies to look into the science of caffeine. Among other aspects, the inquiry will consider cardiovascular and central nervous system responses to caffeine, especially among sensitive groups. It will also consider potential problems due to synergistic or additive effects between caffeine and other ingredients in energy products.

Taylor also emphasized that the food additive process needs to be respected.

"This is about dealing with this proliferation of novel products, used in new ways, delivered to people in ways that could have physiological effects. And our job is not just to stand by and wait and see what happens. We have a law that presupposes that before you do this, you've made a rigorous scientific decision about safety that is either approved by us or generally recognized by other scientists, and we're not there on this stuff," he said, tapping the Monster on the table.

He said that the FDA's food additive policy allows companies to voluntarily inform the agency of the safety of an additive that is not considered GRAS.

"What I found disturbing on this front was that in no case did the companies that are making these decisions about additional uses of added caffeine come to us through that voluntary notification process, and lay the data on the table, and subject themselves to the scrutiny that would come," he told me. "This rigorous exception to the food additive approval regime has evolved into something that has largely stood the system on its head."

So none of the companies making caffeinated energy products—not Coke or Pepsi, not 5-hour Energy or NVE, not Wrigley or Jolt, not Monster, Red Bull, or Rockstar—had asked the FDA's permission to market products with a food additive that is not generally recognized as safe for the products. Taylor's comment cleared up the mystery over why Green Mountain had not been allowed to mix caffeine powder into its K-Cups: It made the mistake of asking if it was OK. The entire energy products industry, worth more than $10 billion annually, has grown without the FDA's explicit approval.

In this way, Taylor said, the companies producing energy drinks and others of the new generation of caffeinated products are not meeting the expectations of the public or the intent of the food additives laws.

"I can't vouch for the safety of energy drinks," he said. "It's not that we can prove them dangerous, but if someone wants us to vouch for them, sorry."

Walking out of FDA headquarters, I passed a display case of the agency's notable efforts. There were packages of DDT and the drug thalidomide. There were a few patent medicines and antique FDA inspectors' badges. The only caffeine was in a bottle of Formula One, one of the ephedra-caffeine blends that had caused heart trouble. I wondered what else the case might hold in twenty years. Maybe some example of caffeinated excess now on the market. Or, more likely, one that is so innovative, so powerful, and so compelling that it has yet to be formulated.

Traveling back to Maine that afternoon, I passed a Starbucks in Reagan National Airport. It was a warm June day, and they were doing a brisk business in Refreshers. But the coffee aroma still wafted from the kiosk, just as alluring as it had been at the Juan Valdez Café in Santa Marta.

And a few hours later, as I drove through China, Maine, the signs out on Route 3 advertised both Pepsi and Coke, products blended with powder from Chinese pharmaceutical plants. I stopped for gas at a country store and found its coolers full of Monsters and Rockstars, and Honest Teas bearing just the merest essence of the brews I'd tasted at Maliandao. Below the register was the standard display of Hershey's bars, looking a long way from Izapa.

The counter next to the cash register was cluttered with energy shots and energy strips. And there, tucked into the front of the display tray for E6 Energy Strips, was a single pack of the Wrigley Alert Energy gum. It was the first I'd seen of the product Wrigley had tried to pull off the shelves. Of course, I bought it. Who knows? It might be worth something someday.

Acknowledgments

My wife, Margot, and daughters, Lila and Romy, were continually supportive throughout this project. They gave me news tips and generally provided ears to the ground, told me when my focus was veering off course or my logic was flawed, and let me know when I was onto a really good story. They are constant sources of inspiration, and I could not have done this without them.

My brothers, Andrew and Charlie, listened patiently and gave me some excellent suggestions, often while biking and skiing, or over coffee. An environmental scientist and a cardiologist, they helped out many times as I tried to make sense of the statistics and the science.

Kathryn Miles and James Redford read parts of the book and provided keen insight and unwavering support. "The Media Personalities" helped out with cold beers at crucial moments. I am also indebted to all of my friends and cousins, and strangers on trains and planes and in coffee shops and bars, who served as litmus tests to see if stories were interesting or mundane.

I was lucky to have landed at Hudson Street Press, where Caroline Sutton gave the book the kind of attention many say has vanished from the publishing industry. Christina Rodriguez did yeoman's work as we moved from draft to final manuscript, scrutinizing the smallest details while keeping the big picture in focus.

Lynn Johnston, my hardworking, insightful agent, believed in this project when few others did. She gently prodded me to improve it and helped to guide it along to its final form.

Thanks to the editors who allowed me to probe into the far corners of the caffeine world, especially Jane Greenhalgh and Andrea de Leon at NPR, Sarah Fallon at *Wired Magazine*, and Luna Shyr at *National Geographic Magazine*.

Reference librarians at the National Archives (in Atlanta and Washington, D.C.) and the Tennessee State Library and Archives patiently helped me to locate buried caffeine arcana. The Belfast Free Library provided sourcebooks and a quiet place to write.

I conducted more than seventy interviews in researching this book, and I have the deepest gratitude for the sources who were so generous with their time.

Thanks, finally, to caffeine, the bitter white powder that inspired this book and provided the focus and stamina to write it.

Notes

Introduction: A Bitter White Powder

x **"There is ample evidence that lower doses":** B. B. Fredholm, K. Bättig, J. Holmén, A. Nehlig, and E. E. Zvartau, "Actions of Caffeine in the Brain with Special Reference to Factors That Contribute to Its Widespread Use," *Pharmacological Reviews* 51, no. 1 (1999): 83–133.

xi **Michael Bedford was at a party:** These details come from the postmortem report conducted by King's Mill Hospital (Post Mortem no. 10H005319) and from "Caffeine Death Sparks Alert by Nottinghamshire Coroner," BBC News Nottingham, October 28, 2010, http://www.bbc.co.uk/news/uk-england-nottinghamshire-11645363.

xiii **Scientists have understood for decades that as little as thirty-two milligrams:** H. J. Smit and P. J. Rogers, "Effects of Low Doses of Caffeine on Cognitive Performance, Mood and Thirst in Low and Higher Caffeine Consumers," *Psychopharmacology* 152, no. 2 (2000): 167–73; H. R. Lieberman, R. J. Wurtman, G. G. Emde, C. Roberts, and I. L. Coviella, "The Effects of Low Doses of Caffeine on Human Performance and Mood," *Psychopharmacology* 92, no. 3 (1987): 308–12.

xiv **One five-ounce cup of coffee:** J. J. Barone and H. R. Roberts, "Caffeine Consumption," *Food and Chemical Toxicology* 34, no. 1 (1996): 119–29; R. R. McCusker, B. A. Goldberger, and E. J. Cone, "Caffeine Content of Specialty Coffees," *Journal of Analytical Toxicology* 27, no. 7 (2003): 520–22.

xiv **Catherine the Great used a pound of coffee:** Katharine Anthony, *Catherine the Great* (New York: Alfred A. Knopf, 1925).

xvi **The two biggest American caffeine stories:** J. C. Busby and S. L. Haley, "Coffee Consumption Over the Last Century," *Amber Waves*, June 2007, http://webarchives.cdlib.org/sw1vh5dg3r/http://ers.usda.gov/Amber Waves/June07/Findings/Coffee2.htm.

xvi **If you put all the Coke ever produced:** Coca-Cola Company, *125 Years of Sharing Happiness: A Short History of the Coca-Cola Company* (Atlanta: Coca-Cola Company, 2011), http://assets.coca-colacompany.com/7b/46/e5be4e7d 43488c2ef43ca1120a15/TCCC_125Years_Booklet_Spreads_Hi.pdf.

Chapter 1: The Cradle of Caffeine Culture

4 **An archaeological dig:** T. G. Powis, W. J. Hurst, M. del Carmen Rodrí-guez, P. Ortíz Ceballos, M. Blake, D. Cheetham, M. D. Coe, and J. G. Hodg-son, "Oldest Chocolate in the New World," *Antiquity* 81, no. 314 (2007).

4 **It is tempting to think:** Much of the background on the history of choc-olate and the origin of the name comes from this readable, authoritative book: Sophie D. Coe and Michael D. Coe, *The True History of Chocolate* (New York: Thames and Hudson, 1996).

4 **They drank it spiked with chili:** You can still see these pitchers at Tapa-chula's excellent Soconusco Archaeological Museum.

5 **A Scharffen Berger 82 percent cacao:** These numbers were in a report titled *Caffeine and Theobromine*, provided by the Hershey Center for Health & Nutrition. You can also approximate caffeine contents based on the chemical analysis by the International Cocoa Organization, which shows that cacao nibs contain approximately 0.7 percent caffeine. As with tea and coffee, the caffeine content in cacao can vary widely.

5 **Hershey, like most mass-market chocolate makers:** This is detailed in federal regulation 21CFR 163.130.

7 **Because it's become so diluted:** Laszlo P. Somogyi, *Caffeine Intake by the U.S. Population* (Silver Spring, MD: Food and Drug Administration, 2010).

8 **Janine Gasco, a California anthropologist:** Among her many writings is this paper showing who benefited from the region's cacao harvest. J. Gasco, "Cacao and Economic Inequality in Colonial Soconusco, Chiapas, Mexico," *Journal of Anthropological Research* 52, no. 4 (1996).

10 **But USDA researchers showed genetic evidence:** J. C. Motamayor, P. Lachenaud, J. W. da Silva e Mota, R. Loor, D. N. Kuhn, J. S. Brown, and R. J. Schnell, "Geographic and Genetic Population Differentiation of the Amazonian Chocolate Tree (*Theobroma cacao* L)," *PLoS One* 3, no. 10 (2008).

11 **The world's cacao harvest:** Organisation for Economic Co-operation and Development, *Atlas on Regional Integration in West Africa* (2007), http://www.oecd.org/swac/publications/39596493.pdf.

11 **African nations produce six times as much cacao:** International Cocoa Organization, *ICCO Quarterly Bulletin of Cocoa Statistics* 39, no. 1 (2013).

11 **The African cacao industry owes:** Tiffany Hsu, "Nestle Promises Action on Ivory Coast Child-Labor Violations," *Los Angeles Times*, June 29, 2012.

14 **In her book about Hershey and Mars:** Joël Glenn Brenner, *The Emperors of Chocolate: Inside the Secret World of Hershey and Mars* (New York: Random House, 1999).

14 **Thomas Gage, the intrepid runaway missionary:** Thomas Gage, *Travels*

in the New World, ed. J. E. S. Thompson (Norman, OK: University of Oklahoma Press, 1958).

Chapter 2: All the Tea in China

16   **By this account, the emperor:** Bennett A. Weinberg and Bonnie K. Bealer, *The World of Caffeine: The Science and Culture of the World's Most Popular Drug* (New York: Routledge, 2002).

16   **Shennong was a productive herbalist:** Alison Mack and Janet Joy, *Marijuana as Medicine? The Science Beyond the Controversy* (Washington, DC: National Academies Press, 2000).

18   **In his 2008 study on tea:** J. M. Chin, M. L. Merves, B. A. Goldberger, A. Sampson-Cone, and E. J. Cone, "Caffeine Content of Brewed Teas," *Journal of Analytical Toxicology* 32, no. 8 (2008): 702–4.

19   **Several recent studies have found that the combination:** C. F. Haskell, D. O. Kennedy, A. L. Milne, K. A. Wesnes, and A. B. Scholey, "The Effects of L-Theanine, Caffeine and Their Combination on Cognition and Mood," *Biological Psychology* 77, no. 2 (2008): 113–22; G. N. Owen, H. Parnell, E. A. de Bruin, and J. A. Rycroft, "The Combined Effects of L-Theanine and Caffeine on Cognitive Performance and Mood," *Nutritional Neuroscience* 11, no. 4 (2008): 193–98.

19   **At high doses:** A. Higashiyama, H. H. Htay, M. Ozeki, L. R. Juneja, and M. P. Kapoor, "Effects of L-Theanine on Attention and Reaction Time Response," *Journal of Functional Foods* 3, no. 3 (2011): 171–78.

19   **Attempting to capitalize:** T. Kakuda, T. Matsuura, Y. Sagesaka, and T. Kawasaki, 1996, "Product and Method for Inhibiting Caffeine Stimulation with Theanine," U.S. Patent 5,501,866, filed March 21, 1995, issued March 26, 1996.

19   **On average, Americans:** Somogyi, *Caffeine Intake by the U.S. Population.*

20   **By legend, Americans' affinity:** Mark Pendergrast, *Uncommon Grounds: The History of Coffee and How It Transformed Our World* (New York: Basic Books, 2010, 2nd ed.).

20   **While the British drink more tea:** E. Fitt, D. Pell, and D. Cole, "Assessing Caffeine Intake in the United Kingdom Diet," *Food Chemistry* 140, no. 3 (2013).

Chapter 3: High on the Mountain

26   **For hundreds of years coffee was used in its raw form:** Pendergrast, *Uncommon Grounds.*

28   **As you might have guessed by now:** David DeSmith, *The 100% Colombian Coffee Book: How Juan Valdez Became a Household Name* (Topsfield, MA: Fort Rowley Books, 1999). Other background on the campaign came from a talk titled "Strategy for Adding Value to Colombian Coffee," by Luis Fernando Samper, of the National Federation of Coffee Growers of Colombia,

delivered February 27, 2010, at the World Coffee Conference in Guatemala City.

29 **A young American journalist:** Hunter S. Thompson, *The Great Shark Hunt* (New York: Summit Books, 1979).

31 **Although Colombian coffee is well-known:** Coffee statistics produced by different researchers and organizations do not consistently agree. Where possible, I have relied on the statistics of the International Coffee Organization, which updates them regularly and makes them freely available to the public.

31 **The industry is worth more than $70 billion:** Martinne Geller and Mihir Dalal, "Analysis: Single-Cup Coffee Sales Seen Growing," Reuters, February 2, 2012.

35 **Inside those containers:** These calculations are based on caffeine content, by weight, of 1.6 percent.

40 **Norton developed a scheme:** Most of the information about the Norton case comes from court filings. See *U.S. v. Michael Norton*, United States District Court, Northern District of California, Case Number CR 96-40173-01-DLJ. See also several news accounts: Tim Golden, "Supplier Is Accused of Selling Cheap Coffee as Top Grade," *New York Times*, November 13, 1996; Peter Fimrite, "Scalding Affidavit on Coffee Fraud/Kona-gate Grinds On, May Spur Regulation," *San Francisco Chronicle*, November 13, 1996.

43 **Goldberger found that the average caffeine concentration:** McCusker, Goldberger, and Cone, "Caffeine Content of Specialty Coffees."

44 **Following in Goldberger's footsteps:** T. W. Crozier, A. Stalmach, M. E. Lean, and A. Crozier, "Espresso Coffees, Caffeine and Chlorogenic Acid Intake: Potential Health Implications," *Food and Function* 3, no. 1 (2013): 30–33.

Chapter 4: Building a Better Cup of Coffee

48 **That was the creation of Green Mountain:** For background on Bob Stiller, see Luisa Kroll, "Entrepreneur of the Year: Java Man," *Forbes*, October 2001. See also the 1998 interview with Michael Gross, "Bob Stiller: EZ Wider Maker, Green Mountain Coffee Roaster, Spiritual Seeker," http://mgross.com/writing/books/the-more-things-change/bonus-chapters/bob-stiller-ez-wider-maker-green-mountain-coffee-roaster-spiritual -seeker/. Information on Green Mountain corporate history was gleaned from company reports, the time line posted to its Web site, and Vermont Senate Resolution S.C.R 52, from April 24, 2008.

51 **This is not a bit of late-breaking news:** *Annual Report of the Secretary of War* (Washington, DC: U.S. Government Printing Office, 1896).

52 **If you'd had the prescience to invest:** Jeff Reeves, "Wall Street's Most Valuable CEOs," MSN Money, September 9, 2011, http://money.msn.com/stock-broker-guided/articleaspx?post=7d710010-3097-4d13-8523

-159dd9598987. This article is one of the many analyses of GMCR stock as it soared in 2011.

54 **The day after his presentation:** Peter Lattman, "An Investor Creates a Tempest in a Coffee Cup," *Dealbook* (blog), *New York Times*, October 17, 2011, http://dealbook.nytimes.com/2011/10/17/an-investor-creates-a-tempest -in-a-coffee-cup/?_r=0.

54 **Soon the Louisiana Municipal Police Employees' Retirement System:** Wilson Ring, "Louisiana Fund Sues Green Mountain Coffee," Associated Press, December 6, 2011.

55 **By Tuesday, they had voted him out:** Candice Choi, "Green Mountain Coffee Founder Explains Sale of His Stock," Associated Press, May 10, 2012.

55 **Stiller has done well by marijuana and coffee:** Joyce Marcel, "Planting a Seed, One Cup at a Time," *Vermont Business Magazine*, July 1, 2007.

Chapter 5: Pulling the Lever

58 **In other words, this is the study:** R. R. Griffiths, G. E. Bigelow, A. Liebson, M. O'Keeffe, D. O'Leary, and N. Russ, "Human Coffee Drinking: Manipulation of Concentration and Caffeine Dose," *Journal of the Experimental Analysis of Behavior* 45, no. 2 (1986): 133–48.

61 **Griffiths and six colleagues:** R. R. Griffiths, S. M. Evans, S. J. Heishman, K. L. Preston, C. A. Sannerud, B. Wolf, and P. P. Woodson, "Low-Dose Caffeine Discrimination in Humans," *Journal of Pharmacology and Experimental Therapeutics* 252, no. 3 (1990): 970–78; R. R. Griffiths, S. M. Evans, S. J. Heishman, K. L. Preston, C. A. Sannerud, B. Wolf, and P. P. Woodson, "Low-Dose Caffeine Physical Dependence in Humans," *Journal of Pharmacology and Experimental Therapeutics* 255, no. 3 (1990): 1123–32.

61 **William Halse Rivers Rivers, a well-born British doctor:** W. H. R. Rivers and H. N. Webber, "The Action of Caffeine on the Capacity for Muscular Work," *Journal of Physiology* 36, no. 1 (1907): 33–47.

64 **Griffiths took that up in a later paper:** L. M. Juliano and R. R. Griffiths, "A Critical Review of Caffeine Withdrawal: Empirical Validation of Symptoms and Signs, Incidence, Severity, and Associated Features," *Psychopharmacology* 176, no. 1 (2004): 1–29.

64 **Carlton Erickson, a University of Texas professor:** Carlton Erickson, "Addicted to Speculation About Caffeine," *Addiction Professional Magazine*, March 1, 2006.

65 **Dr. Sally Satel is also skeptical:** Sally Satel, "Is Caffeine Addictive? A Review of the Literature," *American Journal of Drug and Alcohol Abuse* 32, no. 4 (2006): 493–502.

66 **They recruited ninety-four people who met the criteria:** L. M. Juliano, D. P. Evatt, B. D. Richards, and R. R. Griffiths, "Characterization of Individuals Seeking Treatment for Caffeine Dependence," *Psychology of Addictive Behaviors* 26, no. 4 (2012): 948–54.

68   **According to the Counter Narcotics Police of Afghanistan:** United Nations Office on Drugs and Crime, *World Drug Report 2009* (Blue Ridge Summit, PA: United Nations Publications, 2009).

68   **Caffeine is such a popular cutting agent:** Press Association, "Pair Convicted of Possessing Paracetamol in Legal First," *Guardian*, September 21, 2012.

69   **It's a freebase analogue:** This scary use of caffeine is detailed here: http://boingboing.net/2009/01/19/how-to-make-smokable.html.

69   **It's not quite the cocaine-heroin combination:** L. V. Panlilio, S. Ferré, S. Yasar, E. B. Thorndike, C. W. Schindler, and S. R. Goldberg, "Combined Effects of THC and Caffeine on Working Memory in Rats," *British Journal of Pharmacology* 165, no. 8 (2012): 2529–38.

69   **The most addictive drugs:** N. D. Volkow, J. S. Fowler, G. J. Wang, J. M. Swanson, and F. Telang, "Dopamine in Drug Abuse and Addiction: Results of Imaging Studies and Treatment Implications," *Archives of Neurology* 64, no. 11 (2007): 1575–79.

69   **In a 1997 literature review:** B. E. Garrett and R. R. Griffiths, "The Role of Dopamine in the Behavioral Effects of Caffeine in Animals and Humans," *Pharmacology, Biochemistry, and Behavior* 57, no. 3 (1997): 533–41.

70   **In 1930, the British drugs researcher:** W. E. Dixon, "A Clinical Address on Drug Addiction," *Canadian Medical Association Journal* 23, no. 6 (1930).

70   **In a 2005 literature review:** J. E. James and P. J. Rogers, "Effects of Caffeine on Performance and Mood: Withdrawal Reversal Is the Most Plausible Explanation," *Psychopharmacology* 182, no. 1 (2005): 1–8.

70   **In research published in 2009:** M. A. Addicott and P. J. Laurienti, "A Comparison of the Effects of Caffeine Following Abstinence and Normal Caffeine Use," *Psychopharmacology* 207, no. 3 (2009): 423–31.

71   **In 1996, a British team reported:** N. J. Richardson, P. J. Rogers, and N. A. Elliman, "Conditioned Flavour Preferences Reinforced by Caffeine Consumed After Lunch," *Physiology & Behavior* 60, no. 1 (1996): 257–63.

72   **In a 1981 letter to the FDA:** Letter from Coca-Cola food and drug counsel Michael J. Gilroy to the FDA, July 27, 1981, in reference to Docket No. 80N-0418.

72   **In a 2008 report:** International Food Information Council Foundation, *Caffeine and Health: Clarifying the Controversies* (2008), http://www.foodinsight.org/Content/3147/Caffeine_v8-2.pdf.

72   **Griffiths and a colleague tested cola solutions:** R. R. Griffiths and E. M. Vernotica, "Is Caffeine a Flavoring Agent in Cola Soft Drinks?" *Archives of Family Medicine* 9, no. 8 (2000): 727–34.

73   **The link between obesity and sugary soft drinks:** V. S. Malik, B. M. Popkin, G. A. Bray, J. P. Després, W. C. Willett, and F. B. Hu, "Sugar-Sweetened Beverages and Risk of Metabolic Syndrome and Type 2 Diabetes: A Meta-Analysis," *Diabetes Care* 33, no. 11 (2010): 2477–83.

73   **In 2012, Harvard researchers:** Q. Qi, A. Y. Chu, J. H. Kang, M. K. Jensen, G. C. Curhan, L. R. Pasquale, P. M. Ridker et al., "Sugar-Sweetened Bever-

ages and Genetic Risk of Obesity," *New England Journal of Medicine* 367, no. 15 (2012): 1387–96.

74   **One estimate put the medical costs:** E. A. Finkelstein, J. G. Trogdon, J. W. Cohen, and W. Dietz, "Annual Medical Spending Attributable to Obesity: Payer- and Service-Specific Estimates," *Health Affairs* 28, no. 5 (2009): w822–31.

74   **Kelly Brownell, an expert on food addiction:** Kelly Brownell, interview by Fen Montaigne, "Food Industry Pursues the Strategy of Big Tobacco," *Yale Environment 360*, April 8, 2009.

74–75 **Tobacco industry experts have often made the same point:** J. E. Henningfield, C. A. Rose, and M. Zeller, "Tobacco Industry Litigation Position on Addiction: Continued Dependence on Past Views," *Tobacco Control* 15, suppl. 4 (2006): iv27–36.

75   **Crusading FDA commissioner David Kessler:** D. A. Kessler, "Statement on Nicotine-Containing Cigarettes," *Tobacco Control* 3, no. 2 (1994): 148–58.

76   **The primary trade group:** American Beverage Association Press Office, "Beverage Industry Responds to DAWN Report on Energy Drinks," November 22, 2011, press release, http://www.ameribev.org/news-media/news-releases-statements/more/257/.

Chapter 6: The First Red Bull Was a Coke

79   **In the twenty years:** Mark Pendergrast, *For God, Country & Coca-Cola* (New York: Basic Books, 2013, 3rd ed.).

80   **He was selling more than a million gallons:** Coca-Cola Company, *125 Years of Sharing Happiness*.

80   **"Next week he'll give them mothballs":** Wallace F. Janssen, "The Story of the Laws Behind the Labels," *FDA Consumer*, June 1981.

82   **Things looked bad to Wiley from the start:** Harvey W. Wiley, *Harvey W. Wiley: An Autobiography* (Emmaus, PA: Rodale Books, 1957).

82   **Others testified about the caffeine content:** "Experts Continue to Give Testimony," *Atlanta Constitution*, March 24, 1911.

82   **Testifying for Coca-Cola:** "Experiments Made on 100 Subjects; of This Number of Men 76 Were Not Affected by the Use of Coca-Cola," *Atlanta Constitution*, April 1, 1911.

83   **And some of the testimony was remarkably unprofessional:** "Repudiations from Experts; of Statements Made in Their Own Works," *Atlanta Constitution*, March 28, 1911.

83   **After more established psychologists:** L. T. Benjamin Jr., A. M. Rogers, and A. Rosenbaum, "Coca-Cola, Caffeine, and Mental Deficiency: Harry Hollingworth and the Chattanooga Trial of 1911," *Journal of the History of the Behavioral Sciences* 27, no. 1 (1991): 42–55. Not just this passage, but much of this chapter was informed by the work of Ludy Benjamin, an expert on the works of Harry and Leta Hollingworth. Benjamin's research

and writing have ensured that history will remember these pioneering American psychologists.

87 **Caffeine concentrations have varied:** Samples from 1940 show that Coca-Cola's caffeine content was only slightly lower than it had been in 1909; by 1943, caffeine levels were much lower, perhaps due to wartime scarcity. See February 20, 1981, affidavit of Coca-Cola's Pope Brock and April 13, 1981, affidavit of Lowrie Beacham in Docket No. 1980N-0148.

88 **Hollingworth compiled his research:** Harry Levi Hollingworth, *The Influence of Caffein on Mental and Motor Efficiency* (New York: Archives of Psychology, 1912).

Chapter 7: Hot Caffeine

91 **In 1905, a small chemical company:** Dan Forrestal, *Faith, Hope & $5,000: The Story of Monsanto* (New York: Simon and Schuster, 1977).

92 **By 1921, Monsanto's Levi Cooke:** Committee on Ways and Means, House of Representatives, *Tariff Information, 1921: Schedule A* (Washington, DC: U.S. Government Printing Office, 1921).

96 **Bruce Goldberger and his colleagues found:** R. R. McCusker, B. Fuehrlein, B. A. Goldberger, M. S. Gold, and E. J. Cone, "Caffeine Content of Decaffeinated Coffee," *Journal of Analytical Toxicology* 30, no. 8 (2006): 611–13.

96 **A million pounds sounds like a lot of caffeine:** These statistics were calculated using 2010 sales data from Beverage Digest (http://beverage-digest.com/pdf/top-10_2011.pdf). For example, in 2010, Coca-Cola sold 1,590 million cases of Coke and 927 million cases of Diet Coke. Each case, as the industry calculates it, includes 24 eight-ounce servings. Each eight-ounce serving of Coke contains 23.3 milligrams of caffeine; Diet Coke has 30 milligrams per serving. Put the numbers onto a spreadsheet, and you get 3.5 million pounds of powdered caffeine.

97 **In 1975, soft drinks passed coffee:** Busby and Haley, "Coffee Consumption Over the Last Century."

97 **To meet the needs of bottlers like Coca-Cola:** The United States International Trade Commission provides import statistics for caffeine (commodity number: 2939.30.0000). The ITC does not distinguish between natural and synthetic forms of caffeine.

98 **In a 1942 War Production Board memo:** John Smiley, War Production Board memorandum, November 5, 1942, exhibit V-5 in Docket No. 80N-0418.

98 **According to Mark Pendergrast, in his history of Coca-Cola:** Pendergrast, *For God, Country & Coca-Cola.*

98 **Coke, Pepsi, Dr Pepper, and Royal Crown all reduced:** The reduction in caffeine was cited in a May 10, 1943, letter from FDA commissioner W. G. Campbell to the War Production Board.

99 **The chemist Emil Fischer pioneered the process:** Laylin K. James, *Nobel Laureates in Chemistry, 1901–1992* (New York: John Wiley and Sons, 1993).

99   **The German company Boehringer Ingelheim:** See corporate history online at http://www.boehringer-ingelheim.com/corporate_profile/history /history1.html.

99   **Pfizer was not far behind:** "Pfizer Adds Production Units," *Hartford Courant*, December 11, 1949.

100 **The Pfizer plant mostly stayed out of the news:** "Workers Evacuated at Pfizer Caffeine Unit," *Day* (New London), June 21, 1995.

Chapter 8: China White

105 **We know this courtesy of:** Jay S. Buckley, 1950, "Decreasing Fluorescence of Synthetic Caffeine," U.S. Patent 2,584,839, filed December 4, 1950, issued February 5, 1952.

106 **In 1961, Coca-Cola and Monsanto researchers:** A. B. Allen, "Caffeine Identification: Differentiation of Synthetic and Natural Caffeine," *Journal of Agricultural and Food Chemistry* 9, no. 4 (1961); O. J. Weinkauff, R. W. Radue, R. E. Keller, and H. R. Crane, "Caffeine Evaluation: Identification of Caffeine as Natural or Synthetic," *Journal of Agricultural and Food Chemistry* 9, no. 5 (1961).

106 **Chemist William Knowles:** William S. Knowles, interview by Michael A. Grayson, January 30, 2008 (Philadelphia: Chemical Heritage Foundation, Oral History Transcript 0406).

107 **One flavoring supplier:** The supplier is WILD Flavors, of Erlanger, Kentucky, which provided a list of caffeinated additives in May 2011.

107 **Just three Chinese factories:** This data came from Panjiva, a firm that tracks global trade.

108 **In 2011, Florida Governor Rick Scott:** Jeff Ostrowski, "Brazilian Firm to Open $25M Riviera Beach Site to Make Organic Caffeine, Will Hire 75," *Palm Beach Post*, October 24, 2011.

108 **Picking up where the Coca-Cola and Monsanto:** L. Zhang, D. M. Kujawinski, E. Federherr, T. C. Schmidt, and M. A. Jochmann, "Caffeine in Your Drink: Natural or Synthetic?" *Analytical Chemistry* 84, no. 6 (2012): 2805–10.

109 **A 2007 General Accountability Office report:** See GAO reports: GAO-11-936T, September 14, 2011; GAO-10-961, September 30, 2010; GAO-08-701T, April 22, 2008; and GAO-08-224T, November 1, 2007.

109 **The FDA did make the time to inspect:** See the FDA warning letter WL 320-10-00. The letter from FDA's Richard Friedman, dated May 13, 2010, is addressed to Jilin Shulan president Li DaQian. The FDA placed Jilin Shulan on its Import Alert, or Red List, on January 10, 2011. The FDA resolved the issue with a "close out" letter, dated May 31, 2012. The letter acknowledges that Jilin Shulan addressed the violations. But it appears that by then the company had stopped producing caffeine.

111 **After the inspection:** I retrieved the bills of lading for these shipments from Greatexporters.com, a company that tracks global trade.

111 **When Cadbury Schweppes owned Dr Pepper:** See the annual report *Working Better Together: Our Corporate and Social Responsibility Report 2004*, Cadbury Schweppes Plc External Affairs Department, 25 Berkeley Square, London, W1J 6HB.

Chapter 9: From Stacker to Sunkist

115 **The ephedra problems prompted congressional hearings in 2003:** Commissioner McClellan presented this testimony on July 24, 2003, before the Subcommittees on Commerce, Trade, and Consumer Protection and the Oversight and Investigations House Committee on Energy and Commerce, http://www.fda.gov/NewsEvents/Testimony/ucm115044.htm.

117 **5-hour Energy was selling $1 billion:** Clare O'Connor, "The Mystery Monk Making Billions with 5-Hour Energy," *Forbes*, February 27, 2012.

118 **You might remember the energy drink:** See the FDA warning letter WL 10-07, dated April 4, 2007, and addressed to Redux Beverages.

119 **Scientists studying taste often use caffeine:** For one example, see Susan Schiffman, L. A. Gatlin, E. A. Sattely-Miller, B. G. Graham, S. A. Heiman, W. C. Stagner, and R. P. Erickson, "The Effect of Sweeteners on Bitter Taste in Young and Elderly Subjects," *Brain Research Bulletin 35*, no. 3 (1994): 189–204.

119 **Flavoring houses even sell caffeine-masking agents:** R. Stier, "Masking Bitter Taste of Pharmaceutical Actives," *Drug Delivery Technology* 4, no. 2 (2004): 54.

120 **On September 28, 2010, Robert Callan:** The reporting on this incident came from several dozen pages of correspondence between Dr Pepper Snapple Group and the FDA, obtained through Freedom of Information Act requests.

122 **Another glimpse came just eight months later:** See the FDA recall F-1248-2011, Dr Pepper Snapple Group.

Chapter 10: The Athletes' Favorite Drug

131 **In 1912, several researchers:** I. H. Hyde, C. B. Root, and H. Curl, "A Comparison of the Effects of Breakfast, of No Breakfast, and of Caffeine on Work in an Athlete and a Non-athlete," *American Journal of Physiology* 43, no. 3 (1917): 371–94.

133 **In 2009, Ganio and his colleagues published:** M. S. Ganio, J. F. Klau, D. J. Casa, L. E. Armstrong, and C. M. Maresh, "Effect of Caffeine on Sport-Specific Endurance Performance: A Systematic Review," *Journal of Strength and Conditioning Research* 23, no. 1 (2009): 315–24.

134 **But smaller doses of caffeine can sometimes prove:** G. R. Cox, B. Desbrow, P. G. Montgomery, M. E. Anderson, C. R. Bruce, T. A. Macrides, D. T. Martin et al., "Effect of Different Protocols of Caffeine Intake on Metabolism

and Endurance Performance," *Journal of Applied Physiology* 93, no. 3 (2002): 990–99.

135 **One hydration study followed:** L. E. Armstrong, A. C. Pumerantz, M. W. Roti, D. A. Judelson, G. Watson, J. C. Dias, B. Spokemen et al., "Fluid, Electrolyte, and Renal Indices of Hydration During 11 Days of Controlled Caffeine Consumption," *International Journal of Sport Nutrition and Exercise Metabolism* 15, no. 3 (2005): 252–65.

136 **A group of Australian researchers:** C. Irwin, B. Desbrow, A. Ellis, B. O'Keeffe, G. Grant, and M. Leveritt, "Caffeine Withdrawal and High-Intensity Endurance Cycling Performance," *Journal of Sports Sciences* 29, no. 5 (2011): 509–15.

137 **Alexi Grewal, the American cyclist:** Alexi Grewal, "An Essay by 1984 Olympic Gold Medalist Alexi Grewal," *VeloNews*, April 15, 2008.

138 **American track star Inger Miller:** Steve Herman, "Miller Tests Positive for Caffeine," Associated Press, October 15, 2001.

139 **Taylor Phinney:** Shane Stokes, "Getting the Pill Culture Out of the Sport," *VeloNation*, October 16, 2012.

139 **This is a distinction the American College of Sports Medicine makes:** Lawrence L. Spriet and Terry E. Graham, "Caffeine and Exercise Performance," *ACSM Current Comment*, http://www.acsm.org/docs/current-comments/caffeineandexercise.pdf.

140 **The practice sparked a controversy when England's soccer team:** Dominic Fifield, "Slumbering England Given a Wake-up Call in Poland," *Guardian*, October 17, 2012.

140 **Australian athletes, too, have fallen into this trap:** Nick Mulvenney, "Australian Athletes Handed Sedatives Ban," Reuters, July 3, 2012.

142 **"It's a beautiful theory":** T. E. Graham, J. W. Helge, D. A. MacLean, B. Kiens, and E. A. Richter, "Caffeine Ingestion Does Not Alter Carbohydrate or Fat Metabolism in Human Skeletal Muscle During Exercise," *Journal of Physiology* 529, no. 3 (2000): 837–47.

143 **Tarnopolsky found greater force in the muscles:** M. Tarnopolsky and C. Cupido, "Caffeine Potentiates Low Frequency Skeletal Muscle Force in Habitual and Nonhabitual Caffeine Consumers," *Journal of Applied Physiology* 89, no. 5 (2000): 1719–24.

144 **One dramatic case comes from a musher:** V. Stillner, M. K. Popkin, and C. M. Pierce, "Caffeine-Induced Delirium During Prolonged Competitive Stress," *American Journal of Psychiatry* 135, no. 7 (1978): 855–56.

145 **A group of Australian researchers:** G. Laurence, K. Wallman, and K. Guelfi, "Effects of Caffeine on Time Trial Performance in Sedentary Men," *Journal of Sports Sciences* 30, no. 12 (2012): 1235–40.

Chapter 11: Joe for GIs

147   **That sentence comes from the 1896 Report of the Secretary of War:** *Annual Report of the Secretary of War,* 1896.

151   **Scientists at Walter Reed Army Institute of Research found:** G. H. Kamimori, C. S. Karyekar, R. Otterstetter, D. S. Cox, T. J. Balkin, G. L. Belenky, and N. D. Eddington, "The Rate of Absorption and Relative Bioavailability of Caffeine Administered in Chewing Gum Versus Capsules to Normal Healthy Volunteers," *International Journal of Pharmaceutics* 234, nos. 1–2 (2002): 159–67.

151   **The gum research became:** Mike Dorning and Michael Kilian, "Hastert Sticks Gum Money into the Budget's Fine Print," *Chicago Tribune,* October 14, 1998.

152   **Lieberman is quite familiar with this system:** B. K. Doan, P. A. Hickey, H. R. Lieberman, and J. R. Fischer, "Caffeinated Tube Food Effect on Pilot Performance During a 9-Hour, Simulated Nighttime U-2 Mission," *Aviation, Space, and Environmental Medicine* 77, no. 10 (2006): 1034–40.

153   **Here's how Lieberman described Hell Week:** H. R. Lieberman, W. J. Tharion, B. Shukitt-Hale, K. L. Speckman, and R. Tulley, "Effects of Caffeine, Sleep Loss, and Stress on Cognitive Performance and Mood During U.S. Navy SEAL Training," *Psychopharmacology* 164, no. 3 (2002): 250–61.

156   **A paper from NASA's Ames Research Center:** D. F. Neri, D. F. Dinges, and M. R. Rosekind, *Sustained Carrier Operations: Sleep Loss, Performance, and Fatigue Countermeasures* (Moffet Field, CA: NASA Ames Research Center, 1997).

157   **Army researcher Robin Toblin:** R. Toblin, K. Clarke-Walper, B. C. Kok, M. L. Sipos, and J. L. Thomas, "Energy Drink Consumption and Its Association with Sleep Problems Among U.S. Service Members on a Combat Deployment—Afghanistan, 2010," Centers for Disease Control and Prevention, *Mortality and Morbidity Weekly Report* 61, no. 44 (2012): 895–98.

159   **In one study, Killgore and his colleagues:** W. D. Killgore, G. H. Kamimori, and T. J. Balkin, "Caffeine Protects Against Increased Risk-Taking Propensity During Severe Sleep Deprivation," *Journal of Sleep Research* 20, no. 3 (2011): 395–403.

Chapter 12: Insomnia, Anxiety, and Panic

162   **In 2006, Maryland researchers found:** R. L. Orbeta, M. D. Overpeck, D. Ramcharran, M. D. Kogan, and R. Ledsky, "High Caffeine Intake in Adolescents: Associations with Difficulty Sleeping and Feeling Tired in the Morning," *Journal of Adolescent Health* 38, no. 4 (2006): 451–53.

162   **Wolfson and a colleague found:** A. Bryant Ludden and A. R. Wolfson, "Understanding Adolescent Caffeine Use: Connecting Use Patterns with Expectancies, Reasons, and Sleep," *Health Education & Behavior* 37, no. 3 (2010): 330–42.

162   **Looking at younger caffeine consumers:** W. J. Warzak, S. Evans, M. T. Floress, A. C. Gross, and S. Stoolman, "Caffeine Consumption in Young Children," *Journal of Pediatrics* 158, no. 3 (2011): 508–9.

163   **Caffeine's sleep-disrupting properties:** C. Alford, J. Bhatti, T. Leigh, A. Jamieson, and I. Hindmarch, "Caffeine-Induced Sleep Disruption: Effects on Waking the Following Day and Its Reversal with an Hypnotic," *Human Psychopharmacology: Clinical and Experimental* 11, no. 3 (1996): 185–98.

163   **Swiss scientist Hans-Peter Landolt:** H. P. Landolt, E. Werth, A. A. Borbély, and D. J. Dijk, "Caffeine Intake (200 mg) in the Morning Affects Human Sleep and EEG Power Spectra at Night," *Brain Research* 675, nos. 1–2 (1995): 67–74.

163   **Bedtime reactions to caffeine:** C. L. Drake, C. Jefferson, T. Roehrs, and T. Roth, "Stress-Related Sleep Disturbance and Polysomnographic Response to Caffeine," *Sleep Medicine* 7, no. 7 (2006): 567–72.

163   **A team of California scientists found another variable:** P. Nova, B. Hernandez, A. S. Ptolemy, and J. M. Zeitzer, "Modeling Caffeine Concentrations with the Stanford Caffeine Questionnaire: Preliminary Evidence for an Interaction of Chronotype with the Effects of Caffeine on Sleep," *Sleep Medicine* 13, no. 4 (2012): 362–67.

163   **Even though virtually all of us are aware:** T. Roehrs and T. Roth, "Caffeine: Sleep and Daytime Sleepiness," *Sleep Medicine Reviews* 12, no. 2 (2008): 153–62.

164   **Anxiety itself is remarkably common:** R. C. Kessler, W. T. Chiu, O. Demler, K. R. Merikangas, and E. E. Walters, "Prevalence, Severity, and Comorbidity of 12-Month DSM-IV Disorders in the National Comorbidity Survey Replication," *Archives of General Psychiatry* 62, no. 6 (2005): 617–27.

164   **In a 1974 paper:** J. Greden, "Anxiety or Caffeinism: A Diagnostic Dilemma," *American Journal of Psychiatry* 131, no. 10 (1974): 1089–92.

165   **Greden later looked at how anxiety:** M. A. Lee, O. G. Cameron, and J. F. Greden, "Anxiety and Caffeine Consumption in People with Anxiety Disorders," *Psychiatry Research* 15, no. 3 (1985): 211–17.

166   **In a study of more than four hundred people:** P. J. Rogers, C. Hohoff, S. V. Heatherley, E. L. Mullings, P. J. Maxfield, R. P. Evershed, J. Deckert, and D. J. Nutt, "Association of the Anxiogenic and Alerting Effects of Caffeine with ADORA2A and ADORA1 Polymorphisms and Habitual Level of Caffeine Consumption," *Neuropsychopharmacology* 35, no. 9 (2010): 1973–83.

167   **This is what I call the *Mad Men*:** For a synopsis of the different rates of metabolism and references to the original research, see Fredholm et al., "Actions of Caffeine in the Brain."

167   **This is the primary enzyme:** L. Gu, F. J. Gonzalez, W. Kalow, and B. K. Tang, "Biotransformation of Caffeine, Paraxanthine, Theobromine and Theophylline by cDNA-Expressed Human CYP1A2 and CYP2E1," *Pharmacogenetics* 2, no. 2 (1992): 73–77.

167   **The enzymes essentially reverse:** N. L. Benowitz, P. Jacob III, H. Mayan,

and C. Denaro, "Sympathomimetic Effects of Paraxanthine and Caffeine in Humans," *Clinical Pharmacology and Therapeutics* 58, no. 6 (1995): 684–91.

167   **Strangely, vegetables in your diet can also play a role:** S. Peterson, Y. Schwarz, S. S. Li, L. Li, I. B. King, C. Chen, D. L. Eaton, J. D. Potter, and J. W. Lampe, "CYP1A2, GSTM1, and GSTT1 Polymorphisms and Diet Effects on CYP1A2 Activity in a Crossover Feeding Trial," *Cancer Epidemiology, Biomarkers & Prevention* 18, no. 11 (2009): 3118–25.

168   **In a 2010 literature review, Amy Yang:** A. Yang, A. A. Palmer, and H. de Wit, "Genetics of Caffeine Consumption and Responses to Caffeine," *Psychopharmacology* 211, no. 3 (2010): 245–57.

168   **Writing in the journal *Sleep*:** H. P. Landolt, "'No Thanks, Coffee Keeps Me Awake': Individual Caffeine Sensitivity Depends on ADORA2A Genotype," *Sleep* 35, no. 7 (2012): 899–900.

168   **The A2A receptors Landolt refers:** S. N. Schiffmann, G. Fisone, R. Moresco, R. A. Cunha, and S. Ferré, "Adenosine A2A Receptors and Basal Ganglia Physiology," *Progress in Neurobiology* 83, no. 5 (2007): 277–92.

169   **Nardi was trying to better understand:** A. E. Nardi, F. L. Lopes, A. M. Valença, R. C. Freire, A. B. Veras, V. L. de-Melo-Neto, I. Nascimento et al., "Caffeine Challenge Test in Panic Disorder and Depression with Panic Attacks," *Comprehensive Psychiatry* 48, no. 3 (2007): 257–63.

170   **In another study, Nardi fine-tuned the test:** A. E. Nardi, F. L. Lopes, R. C. Freire, A. B. Veras, I. Nascimento, A. M. Valença, V. L. de-Melo-Neto et al., "Panic Disorder and Social Anxiety Disorder Subtypes in a Caffeine Challenge Test," *Psychiatry Research* 169, no. 2 (2009): 149–53.

171   **In a 1993 letter to:** H. W. Koenigsberg, C. P. Pollak, and J. Fine, "Olfactory Hallucinations After the Infusion of Caffeine During Sleep," *American Journal of Psychiatry* 150, no. 12 (1993): 1897–98.

171   **A case stranger still was reported:** V. G. Masdrakis, G. Vasilios, N. Vaidakis, E. M. Legaki, D. Ploumpidis, Y. G. Papakostas, and C. R. Soldatos, "Letter to the Editor (Case Report)," *Progress in Neuro-Psychopharmacology & Biological Psychiatry* 31, no. 7 (2007): 1539–40.

172   **A team of Australian researchers looked more specifically:** S. F. Crowe, J. Barot, S. Caldow, J. D'Aspromonte, J. Dell'Orso, A. Di Clemente, K. Hanson et al., "The Effect of Caffeine and Stress on Auditory Hallucinations in a Non-Clinical Sample," *Personality and Individual Differences* 50, no. 5 (2011): 626–30.

173   **One case is recounted by Dr. Dawson Hedges:** D. W. Hedges, F. L. Woon, and S. P. Hoopes, "Caffeine-Induced Psychosis," *CNS Spectrums* 14, no. 3 (2009): 127–29.

174   **In Kentucky, Woody Will Smith:** Douglas Stanglin, "Man Accused of Killing His Wife Set to Use a Caffeine Insanity Defense," *USA Today*, September 20, 2010.

174   **Noble's attorney said he had:** Wendy N. Davis, "Killer Buzz: Caffeine Intoxication Is Now Evidence for an Insanity Plea," *ABA Journal*, June 1, 2011.

Chapter 13: Therapeutic Doses

175   **On October 10, 1859, Dr. Henry Fraser Campbell:** H. F. Campbell, "Caffeine as an Antidote to the Poisonous Narcotism of Opium," *Boston Medical and Surgical Journal* 63, no. 5 (1860): 101–4. In this paper, Campbell even described a technique for isolating caffeine. A coffee solution was treated with acetate of lead, "sulpheretted hydrogen" (now known as hydrogen sulfide), and ammonia. The product was pure caffeine: "It presents itself in the form of long, silky needles; is fusible, volatile and soluble in water, alcohol and ether."

176   **One study found that premature infants:** B. Schmidt, R. S. Roberts, P. Davis, L. W. Doyle, K. J. Barrington, A. Ohlsson, A. Solimano, and W. Tin, "Caffeine Therapy for Apnea of Prematurity," *New England Journal of Medicine* 354, no. 20 (2006): 2112–21.

177   **Theophylline, the closely related chemical:** D. J. Henderson-Smart and P. A. Steer, "Caffeine Versus Theophylline for Apnea in Preterm Infants," *Cochrane Database of Systematic Reviews* 1 (2010).

177   **The drug's effects on headaches are complex:** N. Ward, C. Whitney, D. Avery, and D. Dunner, "The Analgesic Effect of Caffeine in Headache," *Pain* 44, no. 2 (1991): 151–55; R. E. Shapiro, "Caffeine and Headaches," *Neurological Sciences* 28, suppl. 2 (2007): S179–83.

177   **Doctors have figured out that the headaches:** M. Fennelly, D. C. Galletly, and G. I. Purdie, "Is Caffeine Withdrawal the Mechanism of Postoperative Headache?" *Anesthesia and Analgesia* 72, no. 4 (1991): 449–53.

177   **But one large study showed that:** R. B. Lipton, W. F. Stewart, R. E. Ryan Jr., J. Saper, S. Silberstein, and F. Sheftell, "Efficacy and Safety of Acetaminophen, Aspirin, and Caffeine in Alleviating Migraine Headache Pain: Three Double-Blind, Randomized, Placebo-Controlled Trials," *Archives of Neurology* 55, no. 2 (1998): 210–17.

179   **For a study published in 2011:** M. Lucas, F. Mirzaei, A. Pan, O. I. Okereke, W. C. Willett, É. J. O'Reilly, K. Koenen, and A. Ascherio, "Coffee, Caffeine, and Risk of Depression Among Women," *Archives of Internal Medicine* 171, no. 17 (2011).

180   **In 2013, Dr. Ascherio and his Harvard colleagues:** M. Lucas, É. J. O'Reilly, A. Pan, F. Mirzaei, W. C. Willett, O. I. Okereke, and A. Ascherio, "Coffee, Caffeine, and Risk of Completed Suicide: Results from Three Prospective Cohorts of American Adults," *The World Journal of Biological Psychiatry* (2013): 1–10.

180   **A 2012 study suggested coffee drinking is linked to longer life:** N. D. Freedman, Y. Park, C. C. Abnet, A. R. Hollenbeck, and R. Sinha, "Association of Coffee Drinking with Total and Cause-Specific Mortality," *New England Journal of Medicine* 366, no. 20 (2012): 1891–904.

181   **Researchers have also found a strong association:** R. M. van Dam and F. B. Hu, "Coffee Consumption and Risk of Type 2 Diabetes: A Systematic Review," *Journal of the American Medical Association* 294, no. 1 (2005): 97–104.

181   **His research showed that caffeine promotes insulin resistance:** T. E. Graham, P. Sathasivam, M. Rowland, N. Marko, F. Greer, and D. Battram, "Caffeine Ingestion Elevates Plasma Insulin Response in Humans During an Oral Glucose Tolerance Test," *Canadian Journal of Physiology and Pharmacology* 79, no. 7 (2001): 559–65; M. S. Beaudoin, B. Allen, G. Mazzetti, P. J. Sullivan, and T. E. Graham, "Caffeine Ingestion Impairs Insulin Sensitivity in a Dose-Dependent Manner in Both Men and Women," *Applied Physiology, Nutrition, and Metabolism* 38, no. 2 (2013): 140–47.

182   **In another surprising finding, Harvard researchers:** F. Song, A. A. Qureshi, and J. Han, "Increased Caffeine Intake Is Associated with Reduced Risk of Basal Cell Carcinoma of the Skin," *Cancer Research* 72, no. 13 (2012): 3282–89.

182   **In an effort to make sense of the studies:** American College of Obstetricians and Gynecologists Committee on Obstetric Practice, "Committee Opinion Number 462: Moderate Caffeine Consumption During Pregnancy" (2010).

183   **But any aspiring mothers who were placated:** V. Sengpiel, E. Elind, J. Bacelis, S. Nilsson, J. Grove, R. Myhre, M. Haugen et al., "Maternal Caffeine Intake During Pregnancy Is Associated with Birth Weight but Not with Gestational Length: Results from a Large Prospective Observational Cohort Study," *BMC Medicine* 11, no. 1 (2013): 42.

183   **Another caffeine quirk:** K. C. Schliep, E. F. Schisterman, S. L. Mumford, A. Z. Pollack, C. Zhang, A. Ye, J. B. Stanford, A. O. Hammoud, C. A. Porucznik, and J. Wactawski-Wende, "Caffeinated Beverage Intake and Reproductive Hormones Among Premenopausal Women in the BioCycle Study," *American Journal of Clinical Nutrition* 95, no. 2 (2012): 488–97.

183   **For years scientists believed that caffeine could contribute:** R. P. Heaney, "Effects of Caffeine on Bone and the Calcium Economy," *Food and Chemical Toxicology* 40, no. 9 (2002): 1263–70.

184   **A 2000 study analyzing data from eight thousand Japanese-American men:** G. W. Ross, R. D. Abbott, H. Petrovitch, D. M. Morens, A. Grandinetti, K. H. Tung, C. M. Tanner et al., "Association of Coffee and Caffeine Intake with the Risk of Parkinson Disease," *Journal of the American Medical Association* 283, no. 20 (2000): 2674–79.

184   **In 2010, a team of researchers from Portugal and Spain:** C. Santos, J. Costa, J. Santos, A. Vaz-Carneiro, and N. Lunet, "Caffeine Intake and Dementia: Systematic Review and Meta-Analysis," *Journal of Alzheimer's Disease* 20, suppl. 1 (2010): S187–204.

184   **Scientists are constantly learning, and even seeing:** D. Elmenhorst, P. T. Meyer, A. Matusch, O. H. Winz, and A. Bauer, "Caffeine Occupancy of Human Cerebral A1 Adenosine Receptors: In Vivo Quantification with 18F-CP-FPX and PET," *Journal of Nuclear Medicine* 53, no. 11 (2012): 1723–29.

185   **More specifically, the traits of introversion and extroversion:** A. P. Smith, "Caffeine, Extraversion and Working Memory," *Journal of Psychopharmacology* 27, no. 1 (2013): 71–76.

186 **Another oddity about caffeine:** L. Dawkins, F. Z. Shahzad, S. S. Ahmed, and C. J. Edmonds, "Expectation of Having Consumed Caffeine Can Improve Performance and Mood," *Appetite* 57, no. 3 (2011): 597–600.

187 **Researchers Valerie Lesk and Stephen Womble:** V. E. Lesk and S. P. Womble, "Caffeine, Priming, and Tip of the Tongue: Evidence for Plasticity in the Phonological System," *Behavioral Neuroscience* 118, no. 3 (2004): 453–61.

Chapter 14: Unleashing the Beasts

191 **In a 1966 regulation defining "soda water":** See "Soda Water; Final Order Promulgating Definition and Standard of Identity," *Federal Register* 31, no. 18 (1966): 1066.

192 **Caffeine ran into trouble in 1978:** For information about the proposal to revoke GRAS status see FDA Docket No. 80N-0418.

193 **After first trying to rewrite the definition:** See "Beverages; Proposal to Repeal Standard of Identity for Soda Water," *Federal Register* 52, no. 97(1987); and final rule in *Federal Register* 54, no. 4 (1989).

194 **The tussle also generated thousands of pages:** K. Szczawinska, E. Ginelli, I. Bartosek, C. Gambazza, and C. Pantarotto, "Caffeine Does Not Bind Covalently to Liver Microsomes from Different Animal Species and to Proteins and DNA from Perfused Rat Liver," *Chemico-Biological Interactions* 34, no. 3 (1981): 345–54.

198 **O'Brien's survey showed that:** M. C. O'Brien, T. P. McCoy, S. D. Rhodes, A. Wagoner, and M. Wolfson, "Caffeinated Cocktails: Energy Drink Consumption, High-Risk Drinking, and Alcohol-Related Consequences Among College Students," *Academic Emergency Medicine* 15, no. 5 (2008): 453–60.

199 **In Gainesville, Bruce Goldberger:** D. L. Thombs, R. J. O'Mara, M. Tsukamoto, M. E. Rossheim, R. M. Weiler, M. L. Merves, and B. A. Goldberger, "Event-Level Analyses of Energy Drink Consumption and Alcohol Intoxication in Bar Patrons," *Addictive Behaviors* 35, no. 4 (2010): 325–30.

200 **In a strange parallel, Buckfast Tonic Wine:** Sarah Lyall, "For Scots, a Scourge Unleashed by a Bottle," *New York Times*, February 3, 2010.

201 **Sales started out slowly:** See McLean Design case study "Creating a Monster," http://www.mclean-design.com/case-studies-type/monster-energy/.

202 **Jennifer Temple, of the University at Buffalo:** J. L. Temple, A. M. Bulkley, L. Briatico, and A. M. Dewey, "Sex Differences in Reinforcing Value of Caffeinated Beverages in Adolescents," *Behavioural Pharmacology* 20, no. 8 (2009): 731–41.

204 **The Portland, Oregon, advertising powerhouse:** Jeremy Mullman, "Wieden Parts Ways with Starbucks," *Advertising Age*, September 23, 2008.

204 **For its part, McDonald's:** Emily Bryson York, "Take Cover! Marketing Blitz for McCafe Is on the Way," *Advertising Age*, May 4, 2009.

204 **Caffeine is also getting plenty of product placement:** Georg Szalai, "Ol-

iver Stone: What Helped Pay for 'Wall Street 2,'" *Hollywood Reporter*, September 29, 2010.

205   **Harris Lieberman and a colleague wrote this:** T. M. McLellan and H. R. Lieberman, "Do Energy Drinks Contain Active Components Other than Caffeine?" *Nutrition Reviews* 70, no. 12 (2012): 730–44.

206   **In the fall of 2012, as lawmakers and regulators:** "5-Hour Energy CEO Discusses Controversial Drink," *CBS Evening News* video, 14:06, November 15, 2012, http://www.cbsnews.com/video/watch/?id=50135243n.

Chapter 15: Behind the Label

208   **In 2011, Arria and Mary Claire O'Brien:** A. M. Arria and M. C. O'Brien, "The 'High' Risk of Energy Drinks," *Journal of the American Medical Association* 305, no. 6 (2011): 600–1.

208   **Around the same time I interviewed:** You can see the ABA document "Guidance for the Responsible Labeling and Marketing of Energy Drinks" here: http://www.ameribev.org/files/339_Energy%20Drink%20Guidelines%20%28final%29.pdf.

210   **Carlson said the FDA produced a document:** "Draft Guidance for Industry: Factors That Distinguish Liquid Dietary Supplements from Beverages, Considerations Regarding Novel Ingredients, and Labeling for Beverages and Other Conventional Foods," U. S. Food and Drug Administration, http://www.fda.gov/Food/GuidanceRegulation/GuidanceDocuments Regulatory-Information/DietarySupplements/ucm196903.htm.

211   **By 2010, caffeine had become controversial in Canada:** N. MacDonald, M. Stanbrook, and P. C. Hébert, "'Caffeinating' Children and Youth," *Canadian Medical Association Journal* 182, no. 15 (2010): 1597.

212   **In 2011, the American Academy of Pediatrics:** Committee on Nutrition and the Council on Sports Medicine and Fitness, "Sports Drinks and Energy Drinks for Children and Adolescents: Are They Appropriate?" *Pediatrics* 127, no. 6 (2011): 1182–89.

212   **The University of New Hampshire wins the award:** This account is based on correspondence I retrieved through New Hampshire's Privacy and Freedom of Information Act.

217   **For adults, ten grams:** P. Nawrot, S. Jordan, J. Eastwood, J. Rotstein, A. Hugenholtz, and M. Feeley, "Effects of Caffeine on Human Health," *Food Additives and Contaminants* 20, no. 1 (2003): 1–30.

218   **Even among those people with arrhythmias:** D. J. Pelchovitz and J. J. Goldberger, "Caffeine and Cardiac Arrhythmias: A Review of the Evidence," *American Journal of Medicine* 124, no. 4 (2011): 284–89.

218   **However, recent research does suggest an association:** M. C. Cornelis, A. El-Sohemy, E. K. Kabagambe, and H. Campos, "Coffee, CYP1A2 Genotype, and Risk of Myocardial Infarction," *Journal of the American Medical Association* 295, no. 10 (2006): 1135–41.

220   **A pair of Arizona neurologists:** S. J. Iyadurai and S. S. Chung, "New-Onset Seizure in Adults: Possible Association with Consumption of Popular Energy Drinks," *Epilepsy & Behavior* 10, no. 3 (2007): 504–8.

220   **Other individual reports of seizures:** R. S. Calabrò, D. Italiano, G. Gervasi, and P. Bramanti, "Single Tonic-Clonic Seizure After Energy Drink Abuse," *Epilepsy & Behavior* 23, no. 3 (2012): 384–85; S. Dikici, A. Saritas, F. H. Besir, A. H. Tasci, and H. Kandis, "Do Energy Drinks Cause Epileptic Seizure and Ischemic Stroke?" *American Journal of Emergency Medicine* 31, no. 1 (2013): 274.

221   **Another strange case comes from Australia:** A. J. Berger and K. Alford, "Cardiac Arrest in a Young Man Following Excess Consumption of Caffeinated 'Energy Drinks,'" *Medical Journal of Australia* 190, no. 1 (2009): 41–43.

223   **When Harris Lieberman and his colleagues:** H. R. Lieberman, T. Stavinoha, S. McGraw, A. White, L. Hadden, and B. P. Marriott, "Caffeine Use Among Active Duty US Army Soldiers," *Journal of the Academy of Nutrition and Dietetics* 112, no. 6 (2012): 902–12.

Chapter 16: Showdown

226   **One problem with caffeinated gum:** Grace Johnson, "School Pupils Sick After Chewing 'Dumped' Gum," *Times Live*, May 12, 2011.

229   **In early 2013, Pepsi launched Kickstart:** PepsiCo, "Discover an Entirely New Way to Do Mornings with Kickstart, an Entirely New Beverage from Mountain Dew," February 11, 2013, press release, http://www.pepsico .com/PressRelease/Discover-An-Entirely-New-Way-To-Do-Mornings -With-Kickstart-An-Entirely-New-Bever02112013.html.

230   **But by 2012, Pepsi was on a roll:** PepsiCo, "PepsiCo's Billion-Dollar Brand Roster Grows to an Impressive 22 Brands," January 26, 2012, press release, http://www.pepsico.com/Story/PepsiCos-billion-dollar-brand-roster -grows-to-an-impressive-22-brands-with-Diet-01262012.html.

231   **In 2013, Coca-Cola posted on its Web site:** The video was produced by Georgia Public Broadcasting for a segment called "Your Health Matters," which is sponsored by Coca-Cola. It was posted online in April 2013 at GPB, http://www.gpb.org/your-health-matters/energy-drinks; and on Coca-Cola's YouTube channel, http://www.youtube.com/watch?v=BBXY 7SDeSHM&list=UU5JBB_E5mzPEbDupD-6fA4A&index=10.

232   **Via is so successful:** Starbucks Coffee Company, "Starbucks to Create More Than 140 U.S. Manufacturing Jobs at State-of-the-Art Plant in Georgia," July 13, 2012, press release, http://news.starbucks.com/article _display.cfm?article_id=679.

236   **Emil Fischer is the German chemist:** Emil Fischer, "Syntheses in the Purine and Sugar Group," in *Nobel Lectures, Chemistry, 1901–1921*, Nobel Foundation (Amsterdam: Elsevier Publishing Company, 1966).

Index